LIVING IN STYLE

INSPIRATION AND ADVICE FOR EVERYDAY GLAMOUR

LIVING IN STYLE

INSPIRATION AND ADVICE FOR EVERYDAY GLAMOUR

RACHEL ZOE

WITH MONICA CORCORAN HAREL

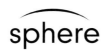

sphere

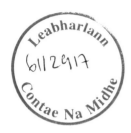

Printed in the United States of America

WOR

First published in Great Britain in 2014 by Sphere

A CIP catalogue record for this book is available from the British Library.

ISBN 978-0-7515-5042-9

Sphere
An imprint of
Little, Brown Book Group
100 Victoria Embankment
London EC4Y 0DY

An Hachette UK Company
www.hachette.co.uk

www.littlebrown.co.uk

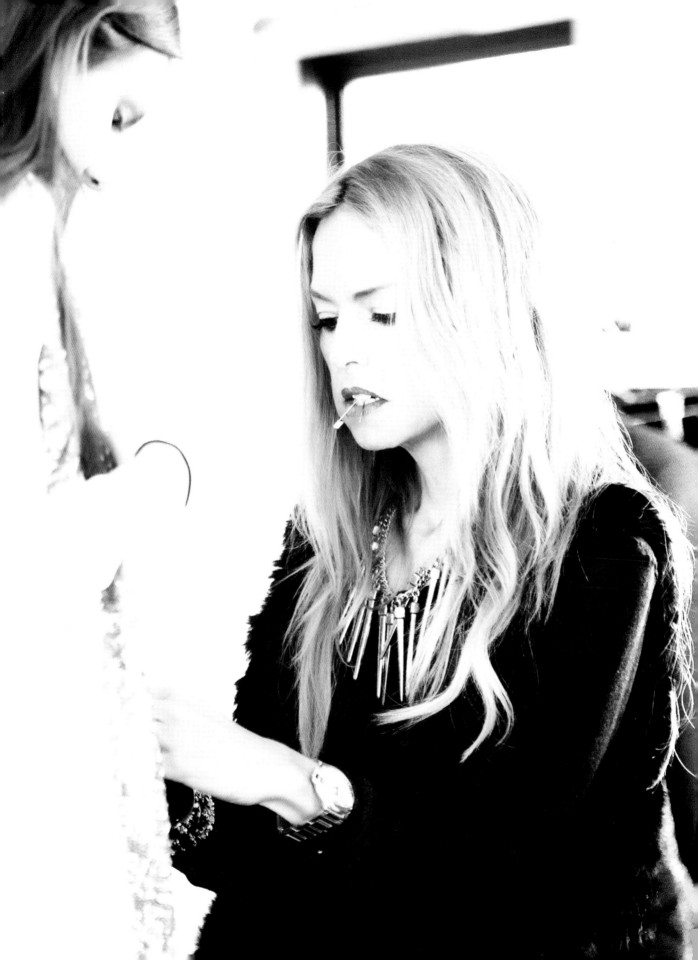

To my idols and mentors, my mother and father; my sister and best friend, Pamela; and my angels, Sophie and Luke. Most of all, to my partner in life and my love, Rodger, and to the light in my life and my heart, my beautiful sons, Skyler Morrison and Kaius Jagger.

CONTENTS

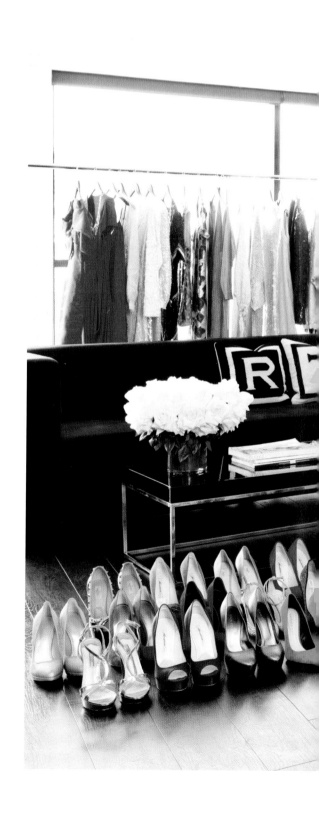

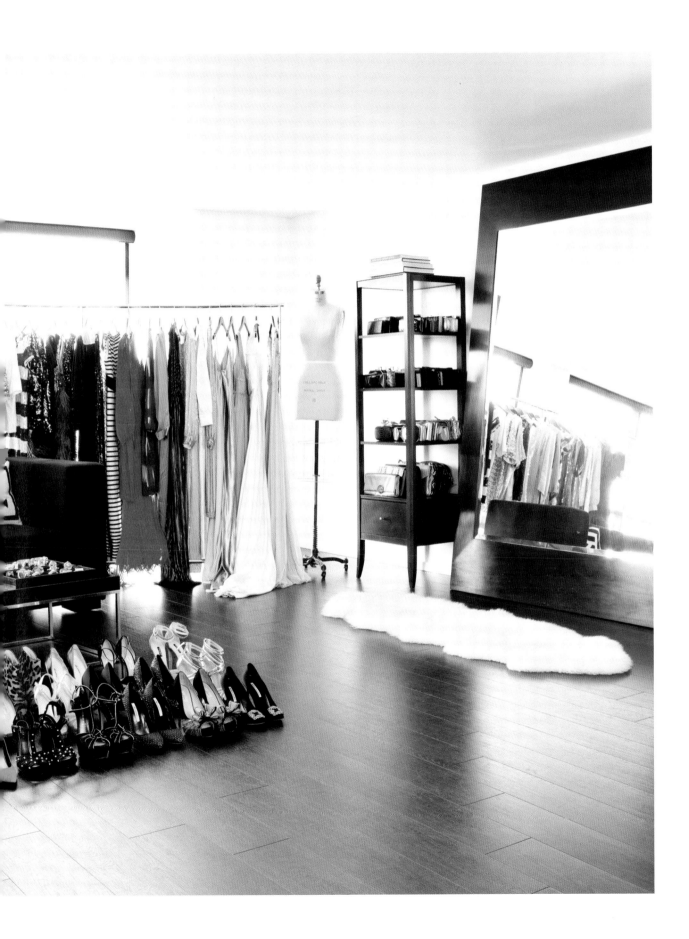

FOREWORD

by Diane von Furstenberg

Everyone wants a glamourous life. To me, glamour isn't just about gold lamé and fancy things. It's shine and confidence. It's a certain independence that comes with experiences that aren't always so glamourous. And sometimes when you look back, those are the moments you value the most. A lifestyle is not just a reflection of what you own or how you travel. It's learning how to create a life that will make you happy.

Rachel loves glamour and she has great taste. She and I first got to know each other when I relaunched my iconic wrap dress about twelve or so years ago. We had lunch in Los Angeles one afternoon and I liked her energy right away. Of course, she and I both share a love for the seventies. But Rachel isn't just my kind of woman because she is chic. She's always on the go and so excited about everything she does. Whenever I see her, she's happy to be part of that particular moment.

That spirit comes through in the way she lives and her talents as both a stylist and a designer. She's a modern woman who listens to the needs of modern women. This book is cleverly broken down to include fashion, beauty, home décor, and family rituals. Let it all inspire you to define your own glamourous life.

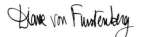

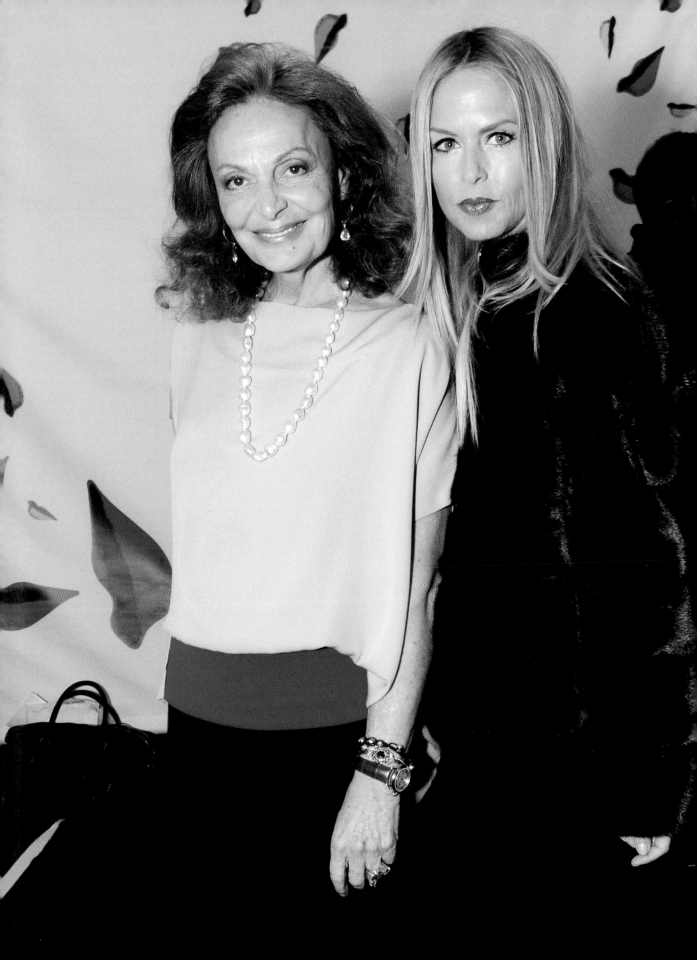

THE NEW GLAMOUR

It's hard to believe that I wrote my first book, *Style A to Zoe: The Art of Fashion, Beauty & Everything Glamour* seven years ago. At that time, as a stylist, my days and nights involved everything from high-profile client fittings to red-carpet premieres to late-night fashion parties. It was frantic, nonstop, and exciting—I definitely didn't get enough sleep! But in hindsight, I now see that I was often focused so much on the details that I forgot to step back and see the big picture. It's not that I didn't realize what an exciting career I had. Believe me, I did. I just rarely slowed down to take a moment and appreciate it all.

> "THERE ARE NO ABSOLUTES IN LIFE. I'LL ALWAYS
> BE THE FIRST ONE TO TELL YOU TO BREAK A STYLE
> RULE—EVEN ONE OF MY OWN."

My life has dramatically shifted since then. Along with being a wife and a stylist, I'm now a fashion designer, a CEO to nearly thirty employees, and a mom to our toddler son, Skyler. You would think that with all this, I would be even more sleep-deprived. Surprisingly, my day-to-day is more manageable now. That's because taking on these new roles and responsibilities has forced me to become extremely efficient—whether it's streamlining my wardrobe to be versatile or reconfiguring my living room for more warmth and comfort. I also had an epiphany along the way. It dawned on me that while my work has always revolved around making people look fantastic (which I truly love to do), I needed to focus on living in style, too. And while my first book focused mostly on the red carpet, the chapters here are a reflection of my own chic world. Since my life evolved dramatically, I've had to redefine some of my own sensibilities and expectations.

Make no mistake—I still love glamour. I will always love glamour. But I have reinvented it in different ways that suit my new lifestyle. My definition of glamour is now a bit more—gasp!—practical. Maybe even a little relaxed, too. And this new outlook applies to everything from my fashion choices to my free time. I now see how denim with a fantastic statement jacket can be as glamourous as a sequined evening dress or why an intimate Sunday supper with friends can be as chic as an over-the-top cocktail party.

What's most important is that I have learned there are no absolutes in life. I'll always be the first one to tell you to break a style rule—even one of my own. I wouldn't be where I am right now if I didn't ignore most conventions and take risks every day.

I'm so excited to share my personal stories, inspirations, and advice with you—not to mention, to help you define glamour in a way that works over time for you, too. It's been twenty years since I started working in fashion. This book feels like a celebration of my two decades in the industry!

CHAPTER 1

FASHION IS MY EVERYTHING

People always ask me how I got my start in fashion. I'll get to that, I promise. But what comes to mind when I think about where my passion for beautiful clothes and my obsession with being a part of this industry began is my very first fashion show. Front row? Please. I literally crashed that runway show. It was Marc Jacobs's spring collection in New York, about fifteen years ago; I had no invitation. In fact, I recall feeling incredible anxiety as I stood in line on the street for hours, not knowing whether I would get in at all.

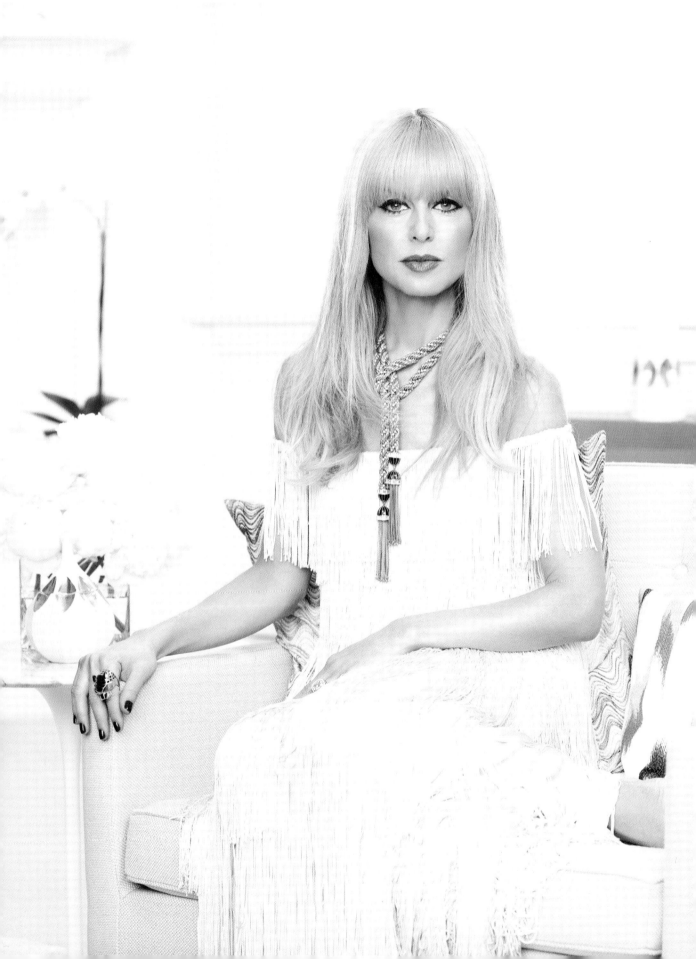

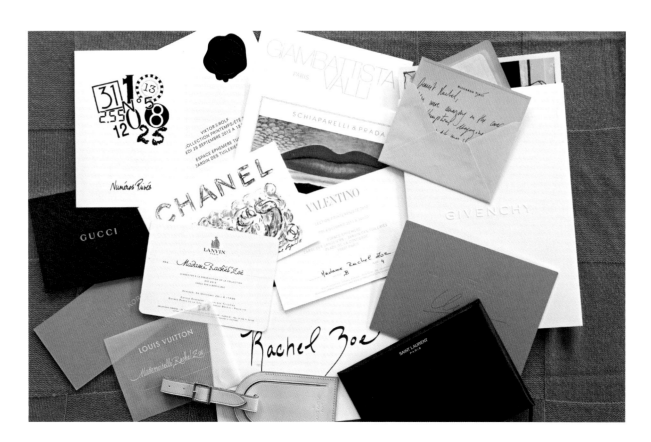

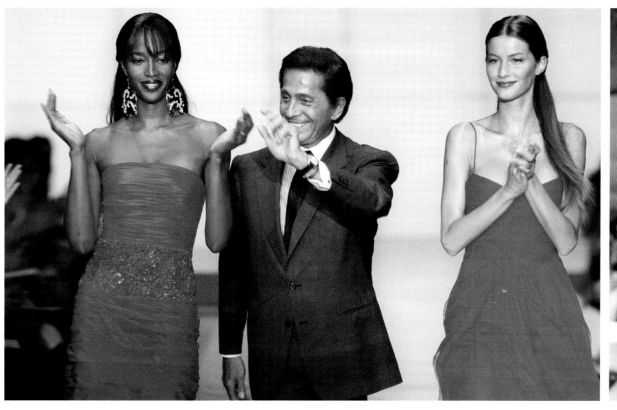

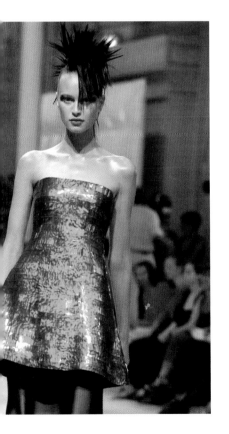

Of course, I can still remember exactly what I wore that day—a vintage black Alaïa dress with six-inch black Manolos. My favorite lipstick at the time was MAC Chili, so my pout was a fiery red. There was no way I was going to miss that show—I was so starry eyed. I would have camped out overnight on the sidewalk, if necessary. A Marc Jacobs show was—and still is—one of the highlights of every Fashion Week. Everyone who was culturally relevant and cool was there, from Sofia Coppola to Winona Ryder, and half of New York wanted a ticket. In my mind, *no* was not an option. A well-known event photographer named Patrick McMullan noticed me lingering outside and snapped my picture—a little black dress can go a long way. He said that he expected to see more of me, which made me feel like I belonged there even more. As soon as the doors opened, I ran to the front and charged through. I even managed to scam a seat, though I was so far back that I couldn't see the looks on the models below the waist. I didn't care.

The runway, the lights, the electricity in the room! I was totally hooked. My next stop *had* to be Paris to see the haute couture shows. I had saved up enough money to finance a weeklong stay in the fashion mecca. "This is my dream. I need to do this," I said to Rodger, who has always supported me. We had just married—I was twenty-six—so I guess you could call the trip my fashion honeymoon. It sounds exciting, but I have to admit I was pretty lonely over there. Working as a freelance stylist in New York, I hadn't yet met a lot of magazine editors or designers. Fashion circles can feel impenetrable.

But once I finagled my way into some of the shows—again, after lots of waiting around and practically begging for tickets—it didn't matter at all. I held my breath as supermodels like Naomi Campbell and Gisele Bündchen paraded down the runways in unbelievable confections of every fabric imaginable. The sheer architecture of Alexander McQueen's collection for Givenchy stunned me. When I glimpsed the elegant, avant-garde gowns and outrageous hairpieces at the Chanel show, my heart literally stopped. Skipped a few beats. Remember your first crush—that rush? For me, this was true love. And I fell hard.

My infatuation wasn't just with the amazing, intricately constructed clothes, though; the fantasy and the glamour and the theatrics made me gasp and even tear up a little. More than anything, the shows reminded me of the transformative power of fashion: you can put on a red dress and take on a whole new identity, or slip into a pair of shoes that alter your horizon in every way.

Even as a little girl, I daydreamed about fashion. I would dash to my mother's closet as soon as I woke up each morning. Who needed cereal and cartoons? I preferred her trove of designer high heels, jewelry, scarves, furs, and jumpsuits. But it wasn't just about playing dress up for me—I didn't even need a mirror. As soon as I layered myself in her chunky tribal necklaces and stood in her chic Maud Frizon heels, I felt instantly like a glamourous woman.

When I was about thirteen, my parents took my older sister, Pamela, and me to Europe for the first time. In Saint-Tropez, I spotted these incredibly elegant women meticulously tanned right down to their ankles and dripping with gold jewelry. Each one of them looked so effortlessly chic, as though she had stepped right off the beach into a little black dress and piled her hair into a messy topknot. Voilà! I knew in that moment that I wanted to be that woman. Always.

And what I realized when we returned home to our traditional suburb of Short Hills, New Jersey, was that I *could* be that woman—well, sort of—if I dressed the part. Pictures from my early teens show me wearing that topknot and as much gold jewelry as I could "borrow" from my mom. Like many others, I also turned to Madonna as my saint of style and sometimes wore rubber bangles up my arms and teased my hair into a wavy bob. All the while, I pored over fashion magazines such as *Vogue, Elle,* and *Harper's Bazaar* for inspiration. I wanted to know everything about new designers and trends. My friends became my models, too. Girls would come to my house after school for their makeovers. I would restyle their clothes with scarves and belts, or roll up their jeans and add new shoes—I even redid their hair and makeup. We called it "Dress up with Rachel."

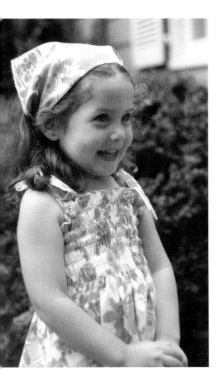

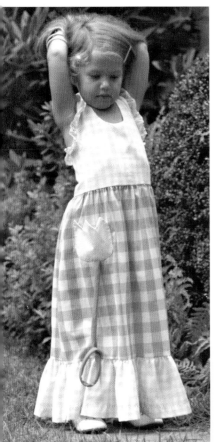

One day, I decided to work my magic on a neighborhood boy who always wore tracksuits. It drove me insane, because his parents dressed so well and I knew that he had fantastic clothes in his closet. I went over to his house and I laid out outfits—Ralph Lauren cable-knit sweaters and khakis to loafers and matching belts—for the entire school week, Monday through Friday. The next day, he showed up looking like he had walked right out of a Polo ad. To see him looking so good made me feel proud and incredibly happy. It was obvious that he felt a whole new sense of confidence.

Back at that time, I had no idea that I could build a career around my love for making people look their best. The closest I came to working in fashion in my teens was a part-time job at Nine West, where I sold the most shoes out of all the employees each week. Even then, I had this contagious enthusiasm for fashion. I would slip a pump onto a woman's foot and say, "This shoe is going to change everything for you." After I graduated high school, I went to George Washington University and majored in psychology and sociology. How we think and behave has always fascinated me; that education has proven to be a great foundation for what I do now.

As a stylist, I understand how fashion can affect your mood and your perspective. It's not *just* about clothes. What you wear is a visual extension of your self-expression. A velvet tuxedo jacket or a vintage caftan can help identify who you are and how you want to be seen. And now, as a designer, I contemplate that power whenever I sketch the strong lines of a suit or test the weight and feel of one of my bold cuffs. Fashion excites me today as much as it did when I sat in the back row and watched that first magical Marc Jacobs show. I still literally get goose bumps when the lights go down and the music starts—whether it's the show of a new and upcoming designer or my own collection coming down the runway.

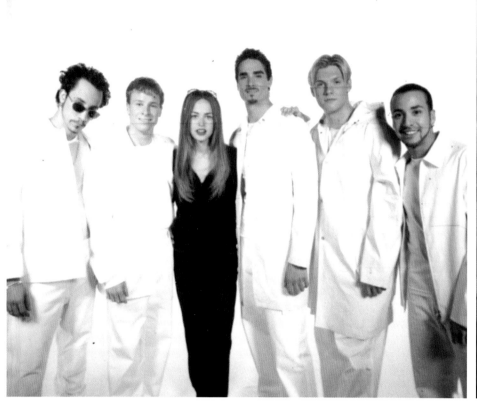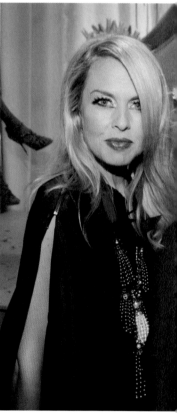

STARTING OUT

Would you rather win the lottery or have dinner with Lanvin designer Alber Elbaz? Does the sight of a vintage architectural Christian Dior cocktail dress from the fifties make your hands shake a little? Me, too. I rarely meet people who are on the fence about fashion and style. Either you love it and breathlessly look forward to the new looks every season or you don't.

My first real foray into this world was styling shoots in New York at the now defunct teen magazine *YM*. At that time, I didn't even realize there was such a thing as a stylist. A friend of a friend told me about a fashion assistant position at the magazine. I was so nervous in the interview, but my obsession with style and designers came through and I got the job. There, I was insanely devoted to making everyone featured in the magazine look chic and cool. I worked long and hard and within two years jumped from assistant to fashion editor to senior fashion editor. The work exhilarated me and I learned so much about the process of creating beautiful looks for editorial covers and photographs. But I also discovered that I wanted to operate more autonomously and creatively. I decided, after two and a half

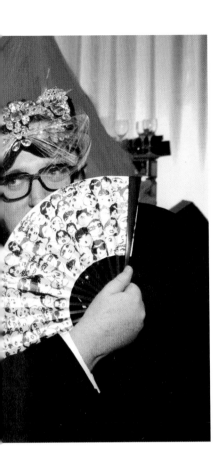

years, to make a huge leap and go out on my own as a freelance stylist. I was terrified, but at the same time, I was lucky that I had such supportive parents and Rodger on my side.

For me, working required a lot of discipline and a lot of faith. Some days, I worked with musical artists like Backstreet Boys, Stone Temple Pilots, and Jessica Simpson. Other days, when I didn't have a gig, I willed my phone to ring with another assignment. Making money wasn't my priority; I was just happy to be doing what I loved on my own terms. I really believe that people who love fashion don't dream of becoming rich—they just thrive on the creativity of the business and fantasize about gorgeous clothes.

In the end, a stylist's job is to make everything look effortless. If you flip through a magazine and skim a fabulous editorial spread, it's easy to assume that the process is as glamourous as those amazing photos, and the same goes for watching a beautiful actress swan down the red carpet in a breathtaking gown. But trust me—a tremendous amount of work precedes those gorgeous fashion moments.

> "PEOPLE WHO LOVE FASHION DON'T DREAM OF BECOMING RICH—THEY JUST THRIVE ON THE CREATIVITY OF THE BUSINESS AND FANTASIZE ABOUT GORGEOUS CLOTHES."

You can't even imagine how many racks of clothes and cartons of shoes and bags get lugged to a photo shoot. I typically call in anywhere from twenty to fifty dresses for an award show; fittings begin about two months ahead of time. It's hard work, no doubt, but I often stop in the middle of a crazy job to take a deep breath and appreciate the wonder of it all, whether I'm choosing which amazing vintage cocktail ring adds pop to a 1960s-inspired photo spread or pinning a couture Chanel gown on an award-nominated actress.

But the true emotional payoff comes when my team and I order in Chinese food to watch the Oscars and I see one of my clients looking ravishing and confident on the red carpet. Later that night, Rodger and I will hit the party circuit and stop by Madonna's legendary after-party. Still now, the chance to be part of such an iconic and glamourous event is always a highlight,

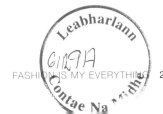

Breaking into fashion is one thing. Climbing up the ladder—in five-inch platforms, no less—requires fanaticism, a great sense of style, and a willingness to learn everything about the business and do anything to prove yourself. Here are my tips for proving that you live (and maybe die a little) for fashion.

BE ABLE TO PRONOUNCE: Azzedine Alaïa (A-zuh-deen Ah-lie-ah), Rochas (Row-shah), Balenciaga (Bah-lehn-see-ah-ga), Givenchy (Gee-von-shee), Rodarte (Row-dar-tay), and Prabal Gurung (Prah-bahl Goo-rung). These and plenty of other designer names will make you stumble. It may require some practice in the mirror, but it's a sign of respect to properly reference someone and not bludgeon a name.

NEVER CARRY: Anything fake. Counterfeit bags with slightly askew logos or mismatched hardware are an affront to designers and editors alike. So much creative thought and hours upon hours of hands-on work go into manufacturing a piece of fashion. Buying a faux anything really is ripping off an artist. If you can't afford a current authentic purse and crave a luxurious designer bag, score a cool, vintage Gucci knapsack or Vuitton bucket bag at a thrift store or an amazing bag without a logo. I love to see someone carrying a unique bag by an up-and-coming designer or a customized satchel that speaks to her own personal style. Your bag should say more about you than just how much you have in your bank account. Be creative in your choice and feel confident about it.

> "MY MOTTO HAS ALWAYS BEEN THIS:
> 'NO TASK IS TOO SMALL.'"

DO CARRY: An emergency style kit that will endear you to everyone, whether you work at a magazine, alongside a stylist, or with a fashion photographer. I keep an SOS kit in my office, too, just in case a colleague snags a dress or spills a latte. The essentials that I always have on hand: safety pins, mini Static Guard spray, travel-sized deodorant, travel-sized lint roller, stain remover pen, wipes, top stick tape, sewing kit, hair elastics or rubber bands, and bobby pins.

DON'T SAY "NO": Making a run for lattes may not be the most glam task, but it will endear you to the VIPs and show some initiative. The same goes for shouldering huge duffels crammed with dozens of ankle boots. My motto has always been this: "No task is too small." Back in the early days, I fetched everything from coffee to packages for a client. On one of my first independent styling jobs, I flew to Monaco alone—for one night!—with six trunks of clothes for Britney Spears. It may have been one of my most difficult and strenuous jobs early on (both mentally and physically), but I felt such pride when I saw her looking so fantastic onstage. I didn't even mind that the customs agents wanted to strangle me.

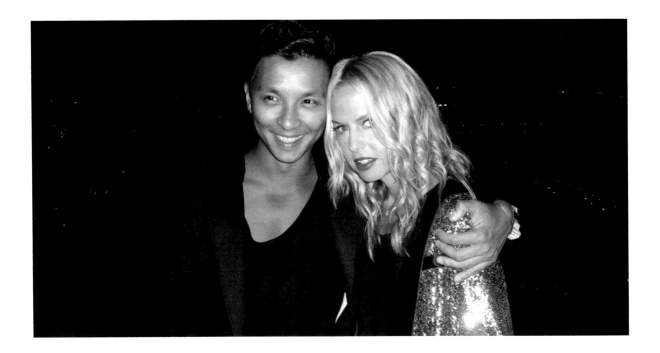

With designer Prabal Gurung

DON'T SAY "YES": If you have agreed to work on a shoot or a fitting and then a better last-minute opportunity arises, pass it up. In a business dominated by trends, fierce loyalty can trump experience and expertise. Fashion is a bit like high school: Word gets around. Plus, the industry is a giant revolving door with editors and publicists and photographers changing jobs frequently. People will remember that you went that extra mile when they move on to a new job. I have worked with the same editors for over fifteen years and still watch them leapfrog from one title to another.

PLAY NICE AND PLAY HARD: Movies such as *The Devil Wears Prada* have depicted the fashion world as a snippy war zone of oversized egos and prickly personalities. Um, that can be true. And I have seen plenty of young people start out with a sense of entitlement that doesn't serve them in the least. In my company, it's the genuinely good and committed people who get ahead. I call my colleagues my "team," because we all pitch in. Important e-mails get answered after hours and on the weekends. We don't worry about whose job it is—or isn't—when something needs to get done. Even I still sometimes do our coffee runs on my way into the office!

ALWAYS HAVE AN ANSWER: When anyone asks me what I seek most in a prospective colleague, my top response is a point of view. I constantly look to my team for their opinion and I value a confident eye. Know your aesthetic, trust it, and speak it. If you have an interview for a fashion assistant position at a magazine or to intern for a designer, be sure to do your homework. I always ask prospective employees to name their favorite designers and to tell me how they stay on top of what's happening in the industry. My advice is to read *WWD*—the daily trade newspaper/bible of fashion—to be in the know. During Fashion Week, be sure to check out all the shows on Style.com so you know what's on trend for the upcoming season.

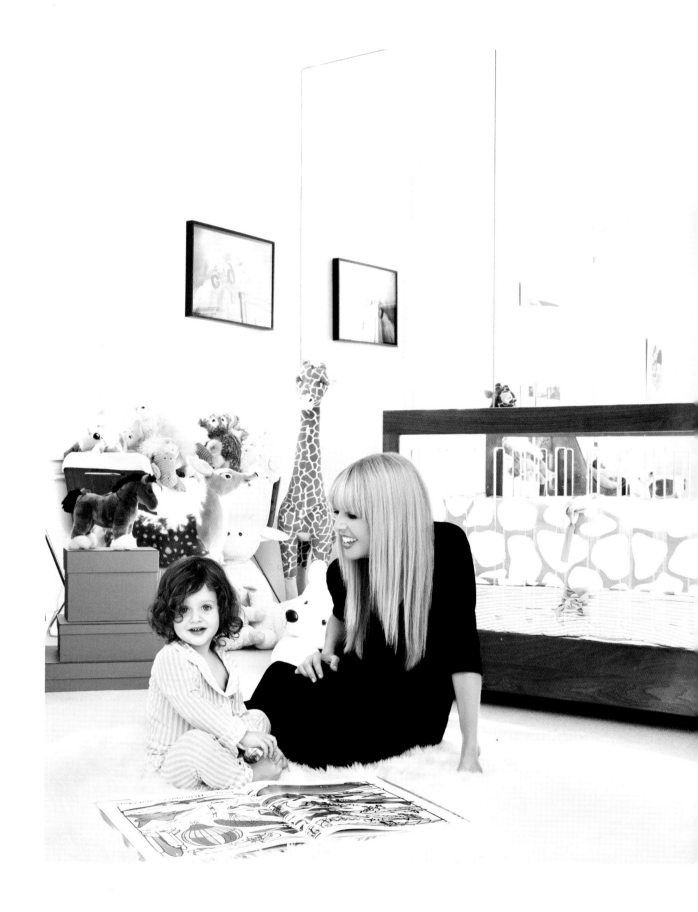

A DAY IN MY LIFE

As a mother, wife, designer, stylist, author, entrepreneur, and obsessive fashion enthusiast, I constantly struggle with the art of balance. There never seems to be enough time in the day to devote myself entirely to each of my passions and responsibilities. Every hour is scheduled with meetings that range from reviewing prototype handbags for my collection to discussing potential partnerships. In the height of award season, I'm dashing to clients' houses for fittings and drinking twice as much tea as my usual three cups a day! But, with all that said, I wouldn't trade any of it for the world. Here is a peek at the schedule I try to keep for the most part, day-to-day.

7:00 A.M.: I wake up and before anything else, go immediately to my son, Skyler, and cover him with morning kisses. Then, I make him breakfast and play with him a bit. That time together is crazy important for me. I like to be with him before Europe and New York start calling.

7:30 A.M.: I'm usually stationed at my kitchen table with a very, very large cup of English breakfast tea and a bowl of berries with Greek yogurt. I get on my computer and begin to filter through my e-mails. I usually wake up to more than a hundred of them—and often, I won't check certain ones before I go to bed the night before, because then I would never fall asleep. In between e-mails I love to skim *WWD* to see what's happening in the world of fashion.

8:30 A.M.: I go upstairs for a three-minute shower and then take thirty minutes to get ready from start to finish—no longer. I typically slip into tailored black trousers or crisp denim with a soft tee and a cashmere duster or structured jacket. I don't lay it all out; I just go by instinct and then grab a pair of heels and sunnies to complete my look. Moisturizer, mascara, concealer, cheek tint, lipstick. A spritz of Tom Ford's Santal Blush and I'm off.

9:30 A.M.: I get into the office, which is always fun, because I love my team so much. First, I check in at the styling studio, which is a floor below my office. I like to work my way up in the building. Together, we skim the racks, discuss past shoots, upcoming editorials, and clients' schedules. We may be pulling for a premiere, a press tour, an editorial shoot, or an ad campaign.

With Skyler

11:00 A.M.: Next, I wander up a floor to meet with my product development office to check if the latest collection samples have arrived yet, or to show them a vintage picture that inspires me. (I get in trouble if I try to sneak by them!) Then, I wander over to my digital team. Typically, I'll meet with the editors of my daily fashion, beauty, and lifestyle website and newsletter, *The Zoe Report,* to discuss upcoming content, trends, likes, and dislikes. I love this part of my day, because I'm surrounded by dozens of twentysomethings who have their fingers on the pulse of everything that has to do with fashion and beauty. It's fascinating to hear about the new street trends and amazing products they discover. After that, I check in with the graphic design team to go over layout and imagery for the website and newsletters. You would be amazed at how much time and effort goes into selecting the size and placement of each headline, border, and image you may breeze over on any given morning. I'm picky…in a good way, of course.

12:30 P.M.: I typically break for lunch around this time, and Sky almost always joins us for the meal. As a mom and my own boss, I'm fortunate to be able to take a little time for lunch each day. Everyone needs what I call a "sanity break," because it gives you clarity when you go back to work. Lunchtime is now one of the most important and satisfying moments in my day—plus, I get to spend some time with Sky! Pre-Sky, lunch was always a walking meal.

1:00 P.M.: On any given day, I might jump right into a footwear sketch review or a resort color and concept preview. During this time, my team and I make edits to the collection while conceptualizing designs for upcoming seasons. I might choose between gold or silver hardware for a bag or examine how a certain fabric falls in a jumpsuit. I love making these creative decisions.

3:30 P.M.: The meetings continue, focused on bigger, broader business issues with the brand and the company. Even though Rodger and I work together, his office is around the corner from mine and we don't visit each other that much. We might walk into a meeting and say "Hi, babe"—but really it's all business during the day. We act like colleagues and always keep it professional. But every once in a while, I like to duck into his office and be a little silly to break up the day. Laughter is very important to me, and I think that's why our nine-to-five relationship works so well. During these larger brand meetings we might discuss prospective partnerships, strategic opportunities, or upcoming appearances at department stores or conferences, which I love to do, because I get to meet the women who wear my clothes.

6:00 P.M.: There are exceptions, of course, but I always try to go home to feed Skyler his dinner. Then later, when Rodger gets home, we give Sky a bath—both of us get splashed—and put him to bed together. Bath time and reading books is a family ritual that brings me so much happiness. Growing up, I remember my mom combing knots out of my hair after bath time and my father singing "Good Night, Ladies" every night to me before bed—until I was thirteen!

7:30 P.M.: In a perfect world, my husband and I sit and have dinner. I order in take-out and we drink a glass of white wine and try not to talk about work. Sometimes we are both in bed by 11:00 p.m. and watch reruns of *Friends* and *Will & Grace* while returning e-mails. But it's more likely that we go out to dinner or have an event three times a week. It's important to make time to support my peers by attending everything from editorial dinners to store openings to product launch parties.

Next spread, left: Fitting a model. Center: Rachel Zoe styling studio. Right: In the design studio.

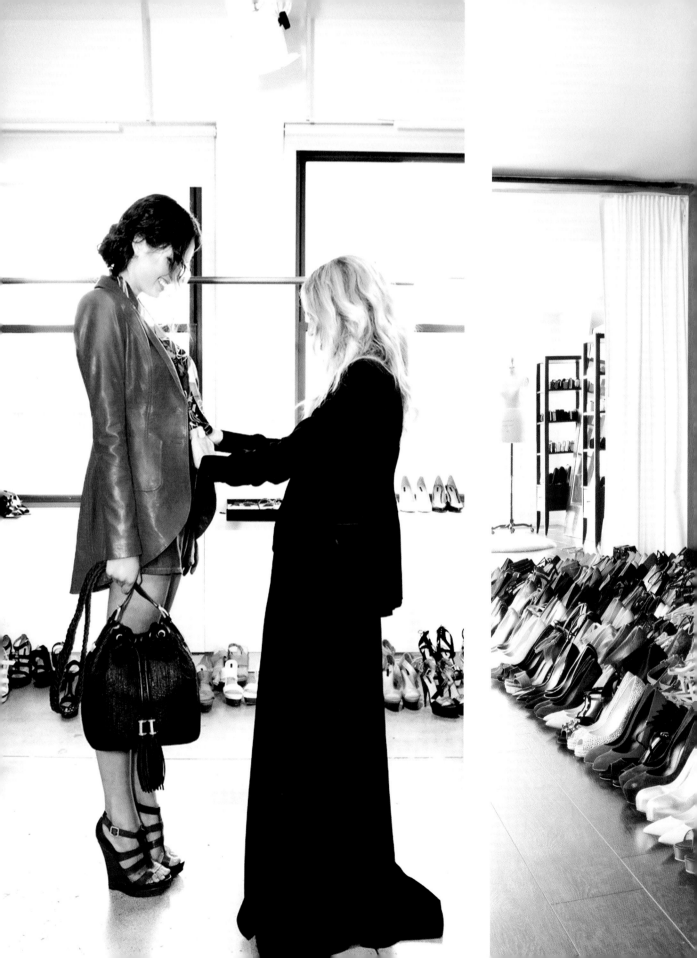

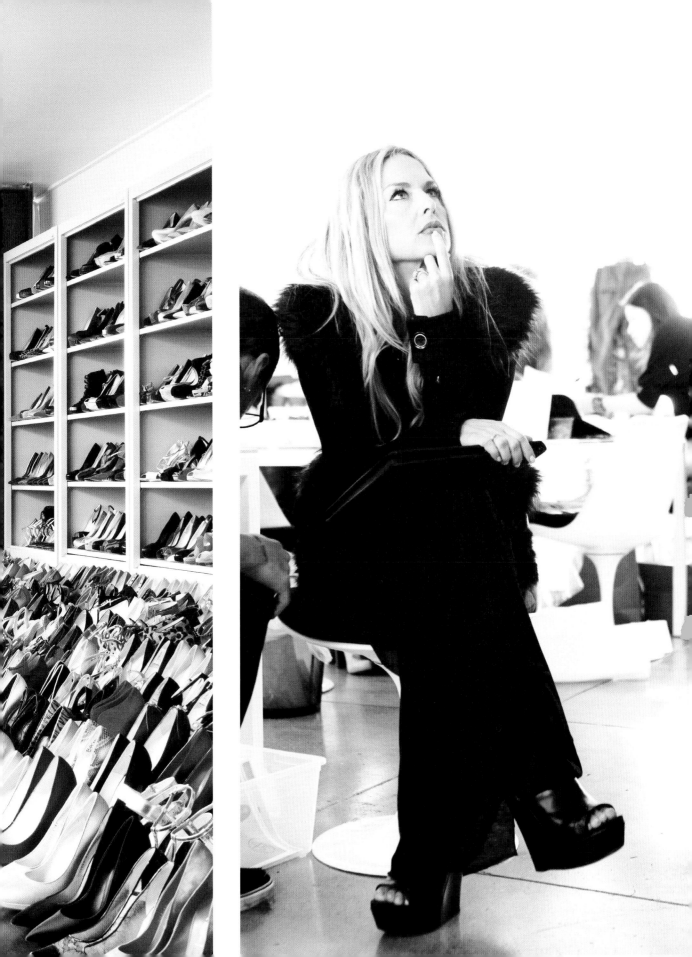

GET IN THE MOOD

Sometimes, the seed of one of my collections is an image. Mick Jagger pouting in a purple velvet slim-cut suit helped me conceptualize my designs for my Fall 2012 looks. Brigitte Bardot frolicking in the South of France with Serge Gainsbourg inspired my dresses for Spring 2013. I will stare at a shot and absorb its spirit—whether it is flirtatious, it has a sense of unbridled sensuality, or something else. It could also be a swatch of caramel leather that piques my creativity. Or a simple stud on a shred of corduroy. In essence, inspiration comes in so many forms, both visual and tactile. So when I sit down to design, I always try to capture the essence of my collection with the help of a mood board. What begins with a few random photos and pieces of fabric might eventually come together as the sensibility and texture of a cropped leather jacket or a pair of pintuck pants.

"WHEN I SIT DOWN TO CONCEPTUALIZE A COLLECTION, MY MIND ALWAYS TIME TRAVELS TO FASHION MOMENTS THAT INSPIRE ME."

Inspiration boards make great starting points for refining your own personal style, too. If you admire Kate Moss's look, tack up a few shots of her in outfits and study her choice of color, silhouettes, and accessories. This can help you focus on the feel and look of an overwhelming event such as a wedding. You don't need fancy supplies to make one—I rely on basic black bulletin boards and clear pushpins, but a blank wall and a roll of tape works in a pinch. There are so many great digital and online tools for making mood boards now, too. And don't be intimidated by a blank one. Nothing is permanent. I post things and then shift them around or replace them all the time. Have fun with it.

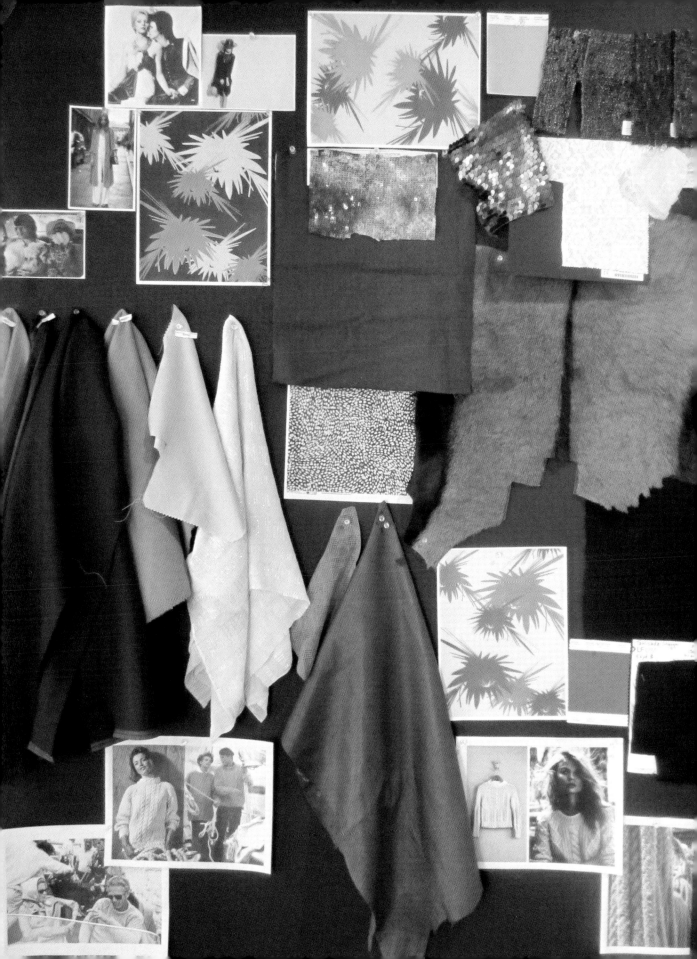

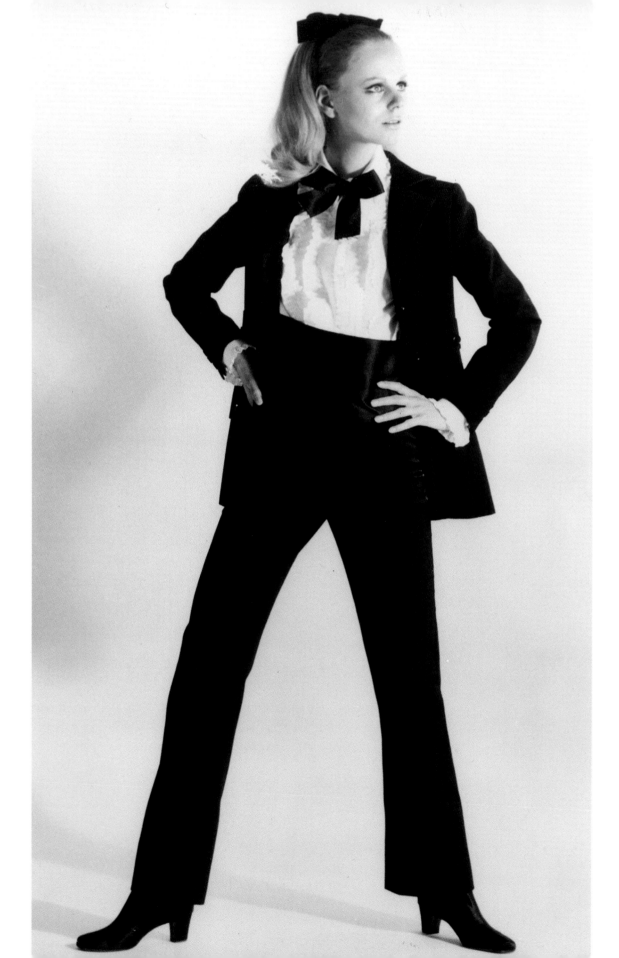

POWERFUL INSPIRATIONS

I'm fascinated by the history of fashion and its standout moments. The silhouettes, fabrics, and even hemlines say so much about the cultural currency of the time. It's no shock that the miniskirt made a splash in the sixties just as women were joining the workforce and reveling in their new-found independence. Mary Quant, reportedly the original designer of the miniskirt, once said that she was inspired to shorten the skirt so girls could run to catch the bus. How cool is that?

When I sit down to conceptualize a collection, my mind always time travels to fashion moments that inspire me. I might reflect on Cristóbal Balenciaga's nod to architecture or Elsa Schiaparelli's passion for whimsy and vibrant color. But you don't need to be a designer to appreciate the past through a prism of style. I often think about a certain decade and its fashion highlights when I get dressed in the morning. If I want to feel particularly empowered, I might think about how a sleek three-piece suit inspired by the late sixties with gold accessories instills me with confidence. Or I might gravitate toward something sequined and off the shoulder that feels more deco as I get ready for a splashy cocktail party. Certain moments in fashion history always influence my personal style and runway collections.

LE SMOKING BY YVES SAINT LAURENT

Catherine Deneuve once said, "The thing about a tuxedo is that it is virile and feminine at the same time." For sure. Yves Saint Laurent's strong-shouldered, formal pantsuit, which debuted in 1966, is always in the back of my mind when I design. It's the most iconic way for a woman to dress, in my opinion. Put on a tux and you suddenly feel strong, confident, and sensual. Like Deneuve observed, it's a unique juxtaposition of the soft and strong.

Make it modern: Go ahead and gender bend. A tailored velvet blazer always looks timeless with great trousers or even denim—high-waisted or skinny. It's an androgynous kind of sexy that reads cool and bold. I love to juxtapose the formality of a tuxedo jacket or trousers with a satin side stripe alongside the casual look of a white tee.

THE BIAS CUT BY VIONNET

This Parisian couturier reinvented sensuality with her mastery of the bias cut: a technique of halving fabric on a diagonal so that it skims every curve of the body. Those 1930s liquid silk gowns worn by screen legends Jean Harlow and Carole Lombard come to mind whenever I think of Madeleine Vionnet, who pinned and draped her dresses on a form instead of sketching designs. She was really the first "body-con" designer—her figure-hugging creations are discreetly sexy as any bandage dress.

Make it modern: I love to juxtapose the proportions of an elegant bias-cut silk chiffon gown with a cropped marabou or faux fur chubby—it's very old Hollywood. Or you can add some street chic to the silhouette with a leather bolero jacket.

THE "NEW LOOK" BY CHRISTIAN DIOR

In February 1947, Christian Dior shocked and awed Paris when he debuted his spring-summer collection. The designer showed accentuated and hourglass silhouettes in decadent fabrics as a tribute to the female form. There were full skirts and jackets with nipped-in peplum waists and sensually rounded shoulders. It was so well received that women attending the fashion show actually mobbed him afterward—and I would have been right there with them. I love the structure in the peplum jackets and the corsetry in the skirts. And I'm always amazed by how he used a form like a figure eight in his clothes to highlight feminine curves.

Make it modern: Every woman should own one blouse or jacket with a peplum waist, which looks great with skinny jeans or a pencil skirt to vary the proportions. I see peplum as a shortcut to looking polished—that cinch instantly delivers a bombshell silhouette. I like to accessorize it with a bold necklace or statement pendant.

THE MISSONI CAFTAN

My dad had a major thing for Missoni sweaters when I was growing up. Every time he went to Italy, he would come home with a new one. I always admired the colorful knits and patterns, but I didn't become a true fan until my first visit to Italy. I saw the scarves and sweaters and caftans and realized that the brand was more about a bohemian lifestyle than it was just about the label. It's amazing to think that this fashion empire began in the early fifties, with the husband and wife founders, Ottavio and Rosita Missoni, creating their own knits. They revolutionized sportswear, inventing that signature zigzag knit on a special machine. I bought my first vintage Missoni caftan when I was nineteen and have since acquired too many to count.

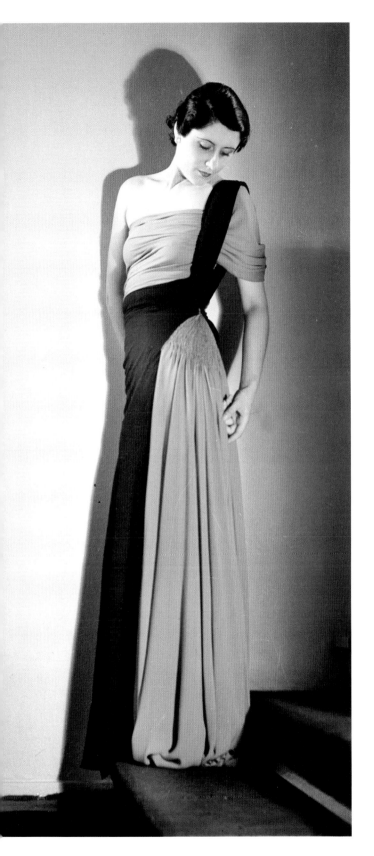

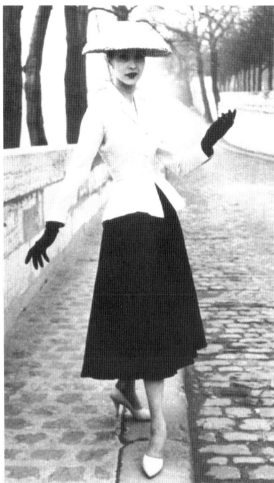

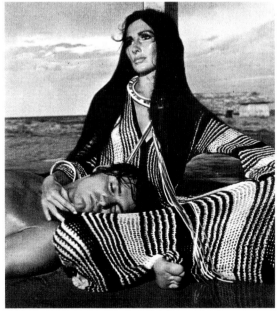

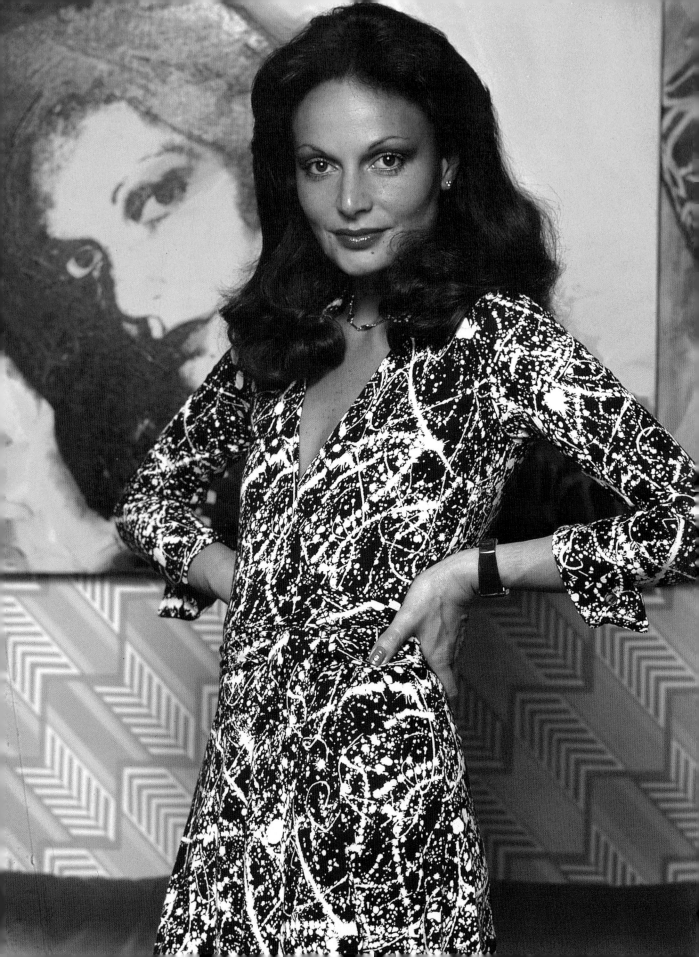

Make it modern: You can spot a Missoni caftan from a mile away—once you get closer, you're intrigued by the intricacies of the knits. I'm not sure how in the world they make some of those unexpected disparate color palettes work, but they always do. I sometimes like to pair mine with a skinny belt or structured jacket to contrast its etherealness. To look a bit more polished, pull your hair into a sleek topknot or wear it down and straight instead of opting for beachy waves or a more tousled style.

THE DIANE VON FURSTENBERG WRAP DRESS

Diane von Furstenberg captured exactly how women wanted to feel in 1972: empowered but at ease. Her jersey knit wrap dress couldn't be more flattering or comfortable. I marvel at the fact that the shoulders are unstructured and yet the silhouette is so strong. This dress looks great on any body type, never wrinkles, and wears as easily as a bathrobe. I also love that DVF once said of her inspiration for the iconic dress: "Well, if you're trying to slip out without waking a sleeping man, zips are a nightmare." That statement in itself epitomized female empowerment at the time of its creation.

Make it modern: The genius of this style of dress is its classic, timeless appeal. You can buy vintage DVF prints from the seventies, which I adore, or you can invest in one of her contemporary versions. I like to wear mine with a stacked wood heel and two bold cuffs on either arm to heighten its power-dress appeal.

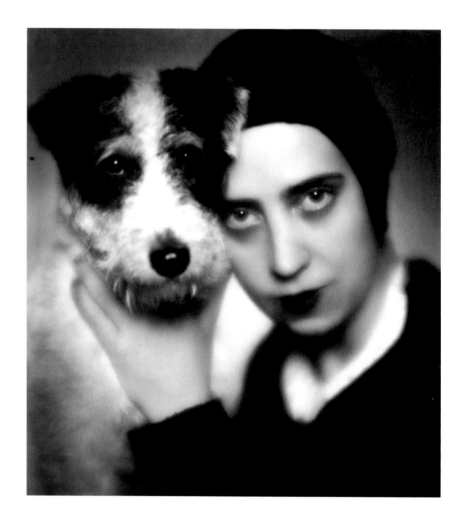

THE TURBAN BY ELSA SCHIAPARELLI

The Italian-born aristocrat had a penchant for shocking avant-garde creations. She was the first one to put zippers on the outside of her designs;
she collaborated with the surrealist Salvador Dalí; and she established hot
pink as her signature color. That's quite a life. She was ahead of her time,
so it's no wonder she also had a thing for turbans, one of my favorite dar-
ing fashion accessories. They just add instant allure to any look.

Make it modern: I love a simple black satin turban with a long white dress
or casual denim worn with a tee and a fitted blazer. The headband version
is the easiest and most current way to wear one. A few years ago, I wore
a satin turban on Thanksgiving and cooked my turkey looking like a 1940s
screen siren. I know it's silly, but why not feel super glamourous while
chopping vegetables? I paid homage to Schiap (as she is known) at the
2012 Metropolitan Museum of Art Costume Ball when I designed a rose-
gold gown and matching turban for model Karolina Kurkova—it was one
of the most surreal moments of my career.

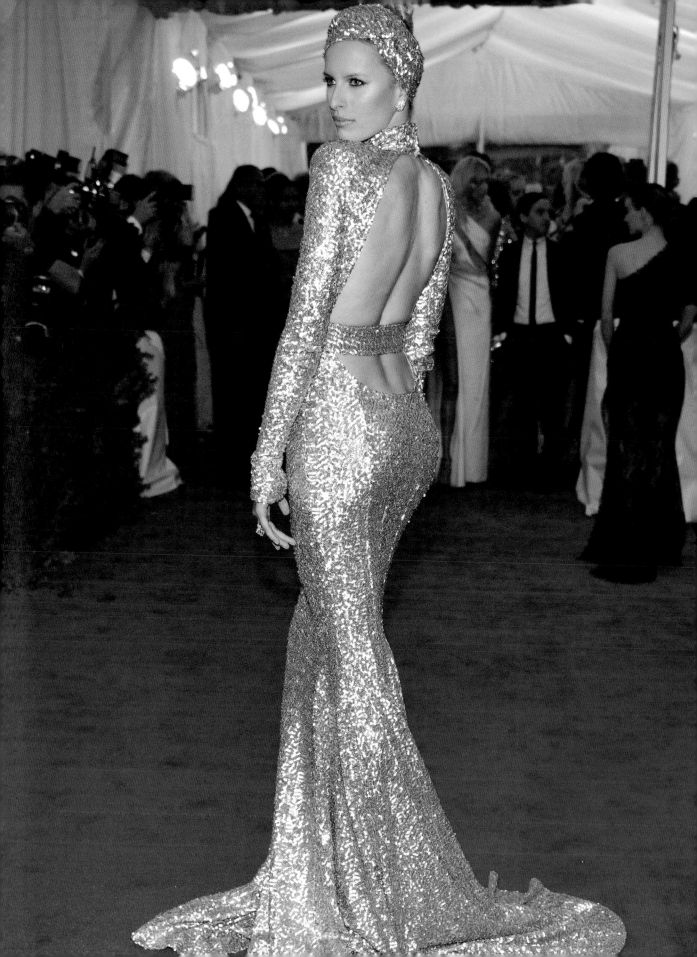

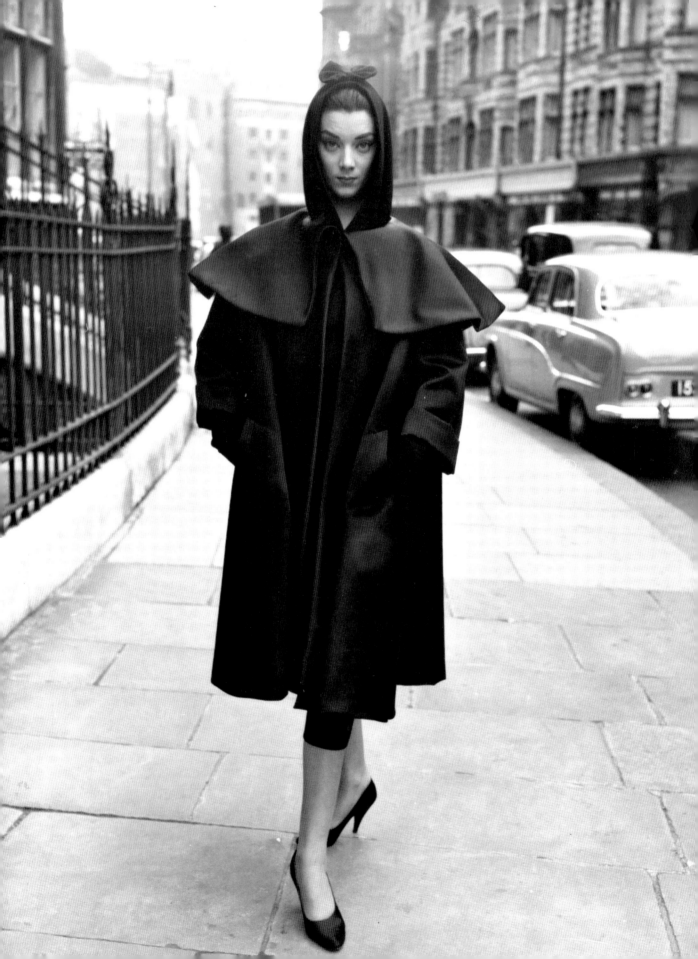

THE COCOON COAT BY CRISTÓBAL BALENCIAGA

Leave it to the genius Spanish couturier to revolutionize proportions and upend the hourglass silhouette with the sack dress, balloon skirt, and my favorite, the 1957 cocoon coat. Thanks to him, geometric forms became fashion. His statement coat with oversized buttons and shorter sleeves allowed a woman to showcase jewelry and elegant leather gloves. The jumbo collar also elongated her neck. Ah, what a difference a few cuts can make!

Make it modern: Oversized silhouettes in outerwear like cocoon coats appear on runways with regularity. I like to see the voluminous shape contrasted with formfitting separates like slim-cut trousers or skinny jeans tucked into knee-high boots. Steer away from pairing the style with an A-line frock, which can swallow you whole and look too retro.

THE ANDRÉ COURRÈGES SPACE AGE COLLECTION

The French designer, who studied civil engineering and favored the architect Le Corbusier, took his cues from technology and futurism in 1964 when he introduced a lunar mission–inspired fashion line. Tunics and minidresses with clean lines, cutouts, and geometric adornments were paired with flat white boots that skimmed the knees. Courrèges made wearing white fashionable all year round, which I believe in, too.

Make it modern: Somehow, the streamlined sixties-inspired dresses and suits still look incredibly modern—fifty years later. The trick to making the styles feel current is to accessorize with on-trend accents like ankle boots or a motorcycle jacket. You don't want to overdo it and emulate all the iconic beauty looks of that era with both pale pink lipstick *and* Twiggy-style over-the-top eyelashes.

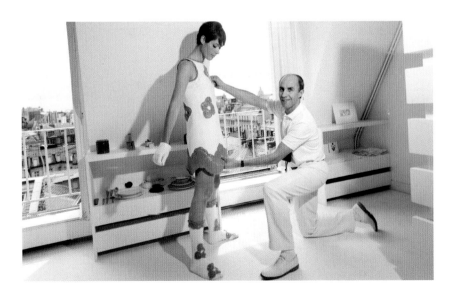

COCO CHANEL'S SUIT

The iconic designer once called her suit "the fashion statement of the century" and I couldn't agree more. She wore her first one in 1910 and at the time, it was a groundbreaking move to challenge the norms of femininity. She even bobbed her hair to further flip off what was socially acceptable for women at that time. When I wear this style, I feel unstoppable. To me, this look is forever. I have said that if I could be known as a designer for great suiting, I would be happy. Every season, I focus on creating these eclectic ensembles that are both classic and current.

Make it modern: The beauty of a well-cut suit — Chanel or otherwise — is that you can wear it thirty different ways. I think it's the best investment a woman can make, in fact. Wear the trousers with a simple silk tank or a sequined top; anchor a flowing day dress or a long caftan with the jacket. You can also pair the jacket with shorts or a miniskirt. It's such a versatile staple.

> "THE BEAUTY OF A WELL-CUT SUIT—CHANEL OR OTHERWISE—IS THAT YOU CAN WEAR IT THIRTY DIFFERENT WAYS. I THINK IT'S THE BEST INVESTMENT A WOMAN CAN MAKE, IN FACT."

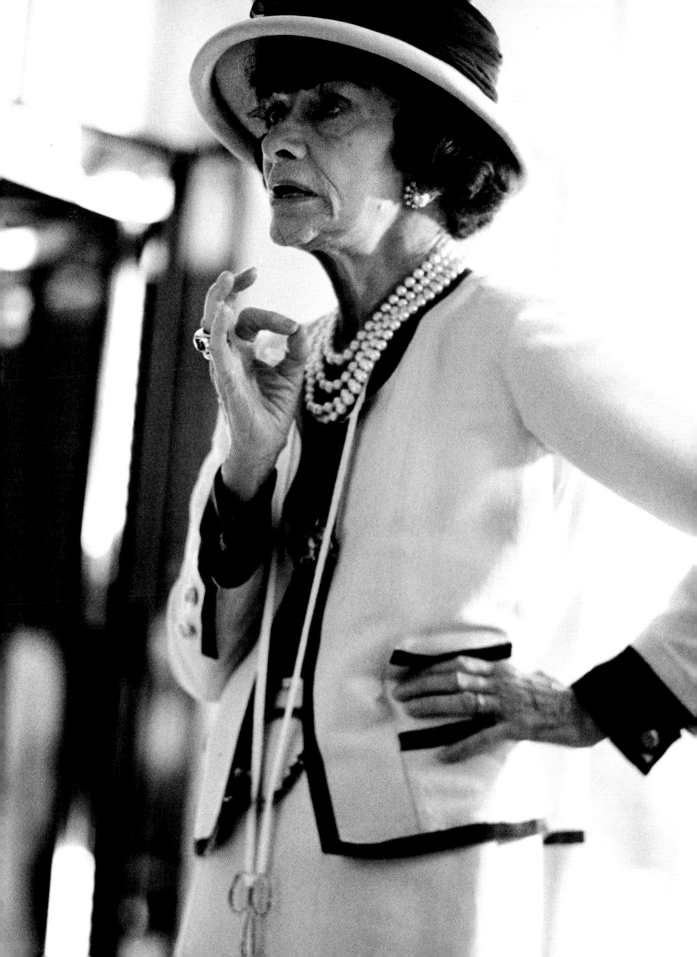

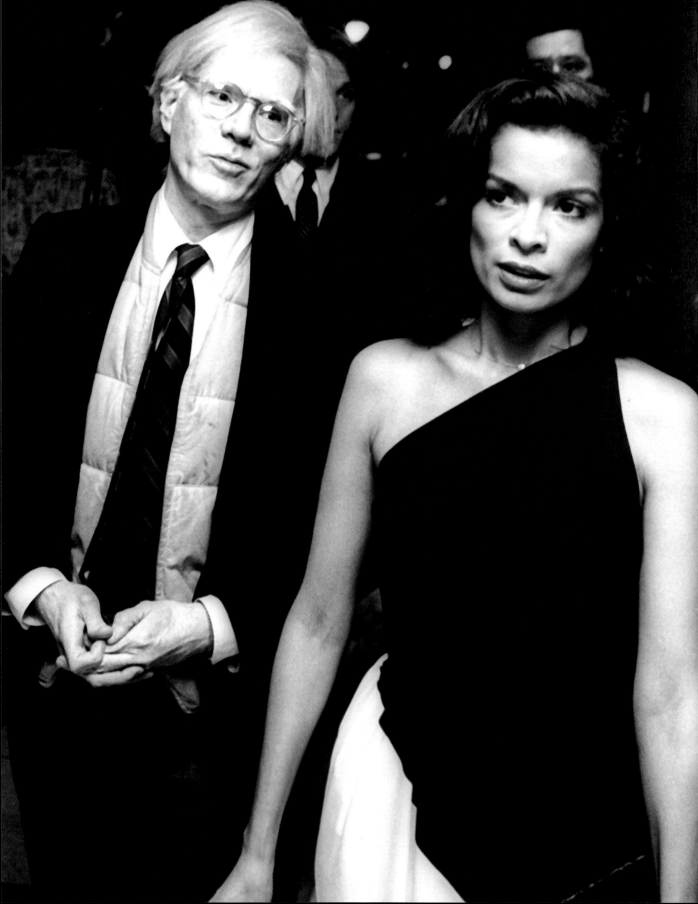

THE MINIMALISTIC GLAMOUR OF HALSTON

At first glance, a Halston design looks so simple. But when you get closer and dissect its construction, you see that it's actually quite complex. To me, that assessment sums up Halston's talent and appeal on so many levels. This man—with his perpetual tan, cashmere turtlenecks, and movie-star smirk—managed to make glamour feel effortless, accessible, and super easy. There's nothing fussy or overly structured about his draped dresses and pleated pantsuits. He understood that women want to look sexy but not distasteful. A Halston one-shoulder jersey dress or cowl back jumpsuit do that perfectly.

Make it modern: Because the designs appear so minimal, I love to pair Halston with bold gold jewelry such as oversized earrings or a collar. Obviously, the pieces are all different, but you can avoid looking like you just left Studio 54 by wearing your hair in a contemporary chignon or side part. But if you want to pay full homage to retro chic, go for it with straight hair parted down the middle and a strappy sandal. I'm such a sucker for that look.

FEAR FACTOR

People often ask me why it took so long for me to launch my eponymous line. My first collection debuted to editors and retailers in spring of 2011 (when I was seven months pregnant) and hit stores that fall. The truth is this: I knew—from consulting with many designers over a dozen years—just how much focus and devotion creating a signature line would entail. Being a designer is a full-time job. I already had a full plate with styling clients such as Anne Hathaway, Kate Hudson, and Jennifer Garner.

> "MY PERSONAL CAREER ADVICE IS THAT FEAR CAN BE A WONDERFUL MOTIVATOR. ONCE YOU FEEL COMPLACENT OR TOO COMFORTABLE, FIND A NEW HURDLE."

And did I mention I was also terrified? Just the idea of putting myself out there gave me emotional hives. I entered this business as a stylist, which kept me behind the scenes. This role reversal meant everyone in the front row would now be critiquing *my* designs. What motivated me, besides my fantastic creative team, was taking on a new challenge. Oscar de la Renta has often told me that he is still nervous before his runway shows—although he appears totally calm. This is a man who trained with Balenciaga and dressed Jackie Kennedy! He said that if he ever stops feeling nervous, it's time to find a new job.

Ironically, just days before that conversation, I had said the very same thing at a conference for fashion and beauty bloggers. My personal career advice is that fear can be a wonderful motivator. Once you feel complacent or too comfortable, find a new hurdle. When I first went out on my own as a stylist, there was no safety net. The hustle was endless, and on days that no work came my way, I channeled my anxiety into drive and ambition. And those same feelings—though in a different context—still motivate me today.

With every collection, I wonder, "Will the editors and critics like it?" and "Will women buy it?" It's not quite a full-on panic, but I can tell you that at times, it's a form of adrenaline that wakes me in the middle of the night with my heart thumping. It also sometimes drives me to act out—like cutting bangs the night before my New York runway show in fall 2012. But in the end, every ounce of anxiety is worth it: I am living my dream. And

I hope that my unconventional path and honesty inspire you, too. Apply for that fashion editor job, launch a style blog, sit down and sketch a ball gown. Remember: If it makes you a little anxious, that's a good thing.

IN EVERY COLLECTION

There has been so much written about building a closet around must-have basics. Fashion editors insist that you should own a navy blazer; friends will tell you that no closet is complete without a pencil skirt. My take? As a new designer, I'm always thinking about the anchors of my collections that work for *every day* and for *forever.*

No matter the season, there are about ten pieces that I will always send down the runway. I strive to make glamorous *wearable* clothes for modern women, whether they're working overtime or jet-setting through time zones. That's my mission. My idea of a basic is a trusted look that works with almost everything—and is anything but basic.

> "I STRIVE TO MAKE GLAMOROUS *WEARABLE* CLOTHES FOR MODERN WOMEN…THAT'S MY MISSION."

SOMETHING SEQUINED: There is no easier way to cheat glamour than with a little sparkle. Sequins don't need to be overly glitzy or precious. They might be leather or suede or even clear paillettes. But I use them in myriad forms and you'll always find a sequined jacket, dress, or blouse in my designs. They go with everything!

CRISP DENIM: Nothing beats a great pair of jeans. I love a denim look that is clean and modern. Find a denim silhouette that works for you—whether it be a skinny- or wide-leg—and dress those jeans up with stilettos and a silk blouse.

A VERSATILE JUMPSUIT: I slip on a one-piece and instantly feel casually elegant. Every one of my collections includes a carefree and relaxed jumpsuit with pockets for keys and a phone, as well as a more structured, sophisticated version. It's my take on loungewear.

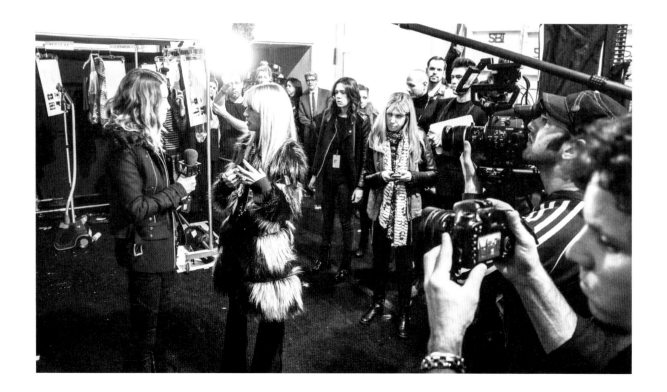

THE LEATHER JACKET: It could be a bomber, a biker, or a blazer, but you should own one for the cool factor alone. Its versatility will astound you once you start experimenting. Wear it with a mini and a tank or even with an evening gown—a contrast I adore. I'm a fiend for all stylish outerwear, whether it's a peacoat or a swing style or a fitted one with military flair such as epaulets. I don't subscribe to the old rule that a coat hem has to exceed that of a dress or skirt beneath it. In fact, a floor-length skirt looks fantastic with a cropped winter coat. One trick I have learned is to wear thin layers underneath so I don't get overheated if I want to keep it on inside.

A TYPE OF TUXEDO: The first piece I ever designed was a double-breasted button-front tuxedo minidress with a notched collar. (I almost did a cartwheel when Jennifer Lopez was later photographed in it.) Dating back to the late 1800s, this tailored formalwear always looks elegant, but modern, too. I particularly like a nontraditional approach, like a tuxedo jumpsuit or dress.

THE WHITE BUTTON-UP SHIRT: I can never get enough of this staple, even though we have seen more than a million incarnations of it. Every season, I design one with a different collar, cuff, or sleeve. This versatile piece looks great with skinny jeans, leather pants, a pencil skirt, and even a maxi skirt.

A CHUNKY KNIT: I think there is a misconception of sweaters being frumpy and conservative. As a designer and stylist, I believe I can make knitwear sexy. That might come across in a sweater dress or a cropped chunky knit worn with a white tank and leggings. I also love an oversized sweater, which can be cozy and luxurious, especially when traveling.

THE THREE-PIECE SUIT: There's a bit of an equestrian and a Victorian feel to this amazing look that takes androgynous femininity to a whole new level. Whether it's a downtown pinstripe skinny suit worn with biker boots or a Park Avenue camel hair ensemble with wide-leg pants, a three-piece suit always looks confident and cool. Best of all, you have great separates to play with.

THE "SURE THING" DRESS: For most women, a no-brainer look is a fit and flare dress that flatters every body type—it gives you a waist and makes your legs look longer. I like one in a neutral tone that you can change up completely with different accessories like boots or lots of metal jewelry or a bolero jacket. Every season, I do a fit and flare and it has become a favorite among my friends.

A MAXI SKIRT: I have lived by this staple for as long as I can remember and I own at least a dozen of them. It's the best way to look glamourous *and* feel comfortable. You never have to be self-aware in a maxi because you are wearing a floor-skimming silhouette that allows you to move freely without being self-conscious about flashing anyone. In essence, it's chic loungewear that looks great with almost everything, from a classic button-down to a slouchy tee to a boyfriend blazer.

I can go on about the art of fashion—from the amazing and pivotal designers to their standout pieces—for hours. But it's the way in which *you* personalize a dress with a bold enamel pendant or a brightly printed scarf that makes it memorable. Yves Saint Laurent once said, "Fashions fade, style is eternal." He knew that even his most exquisite designs called for interpretation by whoever wore them. I couldn't agree more.

When I sketch a suit or a dress, it's just the first step to creating a fantastic look. Even when I see my collection on hangers, it looks incomplete in a way. Why? Because it's up to you to take fashion to a new level by making it your own. Now that we have explored how I became obsessed with beautiful clothes and why certain designers will forever inspire me, it's time to talk about style. Your style.

DEFINE YOUR STYLE

I'm not staring at your shoes. Really. People who don't know me assume that I judge everyone's outfits, from head to toe—not true. In fact, I'm never critical. I appreciate individual style and that has little to do with who can collect the most expensive designer bags or ankle boots. In the art world, you need a ton of money to become a major collector. In fashion, anyone can put together an amazing look—even on a dime. And I love that sense of democracy. All you need is a go-to signature style.

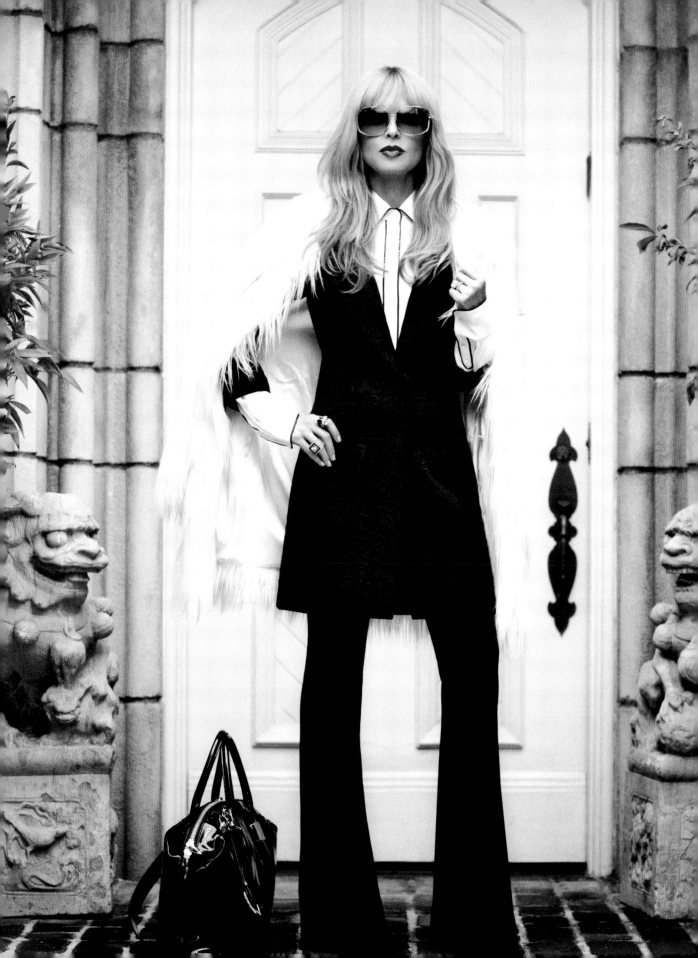

Growing up, my older sister, Pamela, and my mom both unwittingly helped me to shape my style. In my eyes, they were both so effortlessly glamourous. My sister and her friends all ran around in sky-high heels and lots of makeup. My mother, as dramatic in her everyday look as Elizabeth Taylor, never left the house without deep crimson lips and a dozen accessories. She layered sculptural gold necklaces, favored oversized cocktail rings, and wore of-the-moment designers like Norma Kamali and Thierry Mugler. As a little girl with a big personality in suburban New Jersey, all I wanted to do was establish my own personal style like they had, and stand out for it. I still wear many of the accessories that I have "borrowed" from my mom over the years. Her affinity for layering pieces is one of her signatures that became my own, too.

My look was probably at its most creative in my early twenties. I scoured Manhattan thrift stores with a vengeance and experimented with wearing clothes every which way. I often say that the most inventively stylish people I know are the ones on a tight budget. An intern in my office might wear a great vintage locket as a chain belt or a bold ethnic scarf as an obi. I always notice and appreciate that type of ingenuity when it comes to fashion. Never mind a picture—in my opinion, an outfit is worth a thousand words. I encourage you to take some time to evaluate your own look and make sure it's an extension of your personality.

When anyone asks me how to find or even refine her signature style, I offer a few simple suggestions that always help me. Yes, I even reexamine my style now and again to make sure that it suits my current lifestyle. My first tip is to look to anyone whose style you admire. It could be a friend, colleague, sibling, or celebrity. My own look is always grounded in that of the late sixties and early seventies and if I had to name my singular fashion idol from that period, it would be Jane Birkin. (Later on in this chapter, we'll break down her iconic style.)

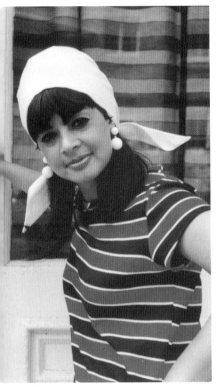

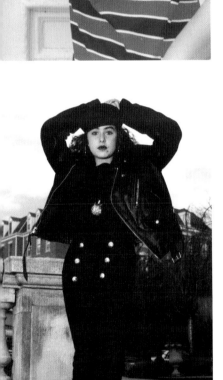

Be sure to immerse yourself in your icon's style. Look for pictures of her online if she is famous and peruse her fashion habits. If your icon is a friend, ask her to define her personal style and even tour her closet. Does she wear a lot of bohemian peasant tops with skinny jeans and equestrian boots? Or is she more polished, in herringbone suits with silk chiffon blouses and platform pumps? Either way, after you take notes on her nuances, you can look to see if you have similar pieces in your own wardrobe. It's so much easier to shop once you know exactly what you need!

Figure out your fashion comfort zone. Every woman I know and client I style has an excess of one thing in her closet. You do, too, no doubt. Look at your own clothes and see which piece or pieces dominate. If my closet could talk, it would scream "Stop buying jackets, Rachel!" But I can't help myself! Tailored jackets are my happy place. And more important, they work for me. You need to determine if your staple does the same for you. If you have a surplus of chunky knit cardigans or pencil skirts, you can assume that these pieces comprise that sartorial comfort zone. We tend to buy the same piece over and over—in different shades and fabrics—because it's safe and familiar. Hopefully, these particular items are major assets to your style.

One easy way to find out is to do this: Try on a few of them in front of a full-length mirror and truthfully assess how they look on you from every angle. Take pictures so that you can be as objective as possible. Be sure to pair them with a number of other pieces to gauge how they work within your daily wardrobe. You should also access how you feel emotionally when you wear these clothes. If you're hiding under oversized sweaters, you probably broadcast insecurity when you wear them; it might be time to experiment with tops that accentuate your natural silhouette and *don't* swallow you up. If you put on a pencil skirt and immediately feel like you can ask for a promotion, that's a powerful piece in your fashion arsenal and one you should keep.

Trust your instincts, but don't be afraid to ask a friend or a spouse to step in as reinforcement. Just make sure it's someone who has great taste and won't be too harsh in the critique. When I'm on the fence about my outfit, I turn to Rodger. Let's face it: I've been with this man for more than twenty years and he knows me better than anyone. So much of looking fantastic comes from feeling truly confident in your look. Rodger can tell in a second if I'm pulling on the bodice of a vintage silk dress or tugging at the sleeves of a knit caftan. He knows from my anxious pout and furrowed brow if I want to turn around and change. So I trust him when he tells me I look unforgettable or uncomfortable. Then again, there are times when he scratches his head at one of my fashion-forward getups and I say, "Babe, this is a fashion thing and I don't need a straight man's opinion. I'm not trying to look hot today."

My final tip for developing your individual style involves a little word play. Think of an adjective—or even a few—that describes how you want to look and feel. *Glamourous* is always on the forefront of my mind when I get dressed. That doesn't mean I walk out the door every morning in Grecian-inspired Halston gowns and faux fur stoles. I also want to look and feel *effortless* and *strong*. For me, these words don't need to be translated literally with specific pieces. They more summon the spirit of my style. I might access *glamourous* with one of the bold deco-chic cuffs I designed with enamel, jade, and pavé rhinestones. Once I slip it on, I immediately feel more cosmopolitan. I get to *effortless* by wearing my hair in loose Brigitte Bardot–esque waves or throwing a tuxedo jacket over my shoulders. *Strong* might come from an oversized structured bag or a tailored suit. You can also think about how you would want someone else to describe your style in a few choice words. If *polished* and *classic* come to mind, go for timeless pieces like wool crepe day dresses and silk chiffon blouses. Craving a *bohemian* aura? Think about amassing printed maxi dresses, caftans, and silk-gauze wide-leg pants.

Once you have your look down, you can build a wardrobe that embodies your signature style—and also edit out the pieces that don't complement your fashion personae. The major payoff to cultivating your signature style is the confidence you feel because your look says it all: "This is who I am."

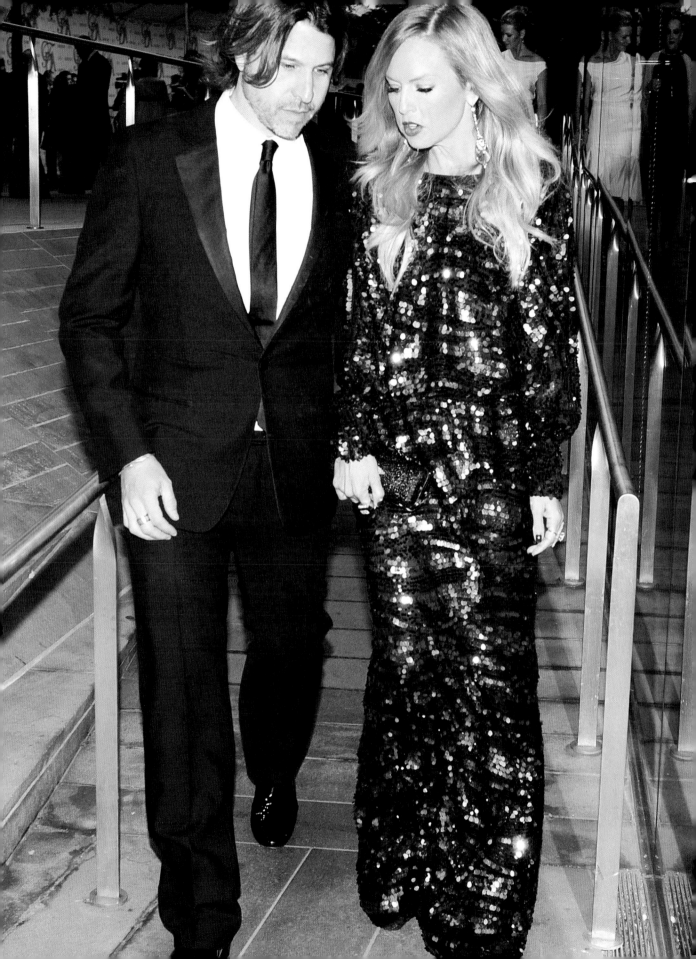

In Wolford tights, Paris
Fashion Week, 2011

ACCENTUATE WHAT'S GREAT

Coco Chanel once said that showing your knees was "hardly ever pretty." (I love it when my all-time idol and I think alike!) I don't like my knees. I can't even pinpoint why, exactly, except to say that they look a little chickeny. In fact, you won't find a recent picture of me in shorts or a minidress unless I'm also wearing opaque tights. Rationally, I know that my joints are totally normal, of course. But the reality is that I am uncomfortable when I expose them. So I don't.

Instead, I dress to highlight my upper body, thanks to a long torso, defined, feminine shoulders, and an elongated neck. I showcase these favorite features by wearing open necklines and off-the-shoulder dresses or tanks. Long necklaces also give the illusion of extending the upper body. Once you know which areas you want to accentuate, focus on necklines, silhouettes, sleeves, and hemlines that do just that. Fashion is a lot like magic, and over years of styling dozens of women, I have developed more than a few tricks for highlighting your best features.

GIVE AN INCH: When it comes to hemlines, even a half-inch alteration can extend the line of the leg. Experiment with the length of a skirt or dress to see where your hem falls best. Just above or below the knee is usually the sweet spot, but trust your eye and instinct.

THE PRICE OF GOLD (AND SILVER): As much as I adore metallic fabrics, their reflective quality can make you appear larger if you have va-va-voom curves. By the same token, that effect may be something you're going for, depending on your body type. Examine how light hits a metallic dress or consider a separate such as gold lamé capri pants or a silver sequined top.

CINCH EFFECT: If you want your torso to appear longer, wear a belt on the lowest point of your natural waistline. Or, a wide belt worn a little higher than your waist always creates more of a classic hourglass silhouette.

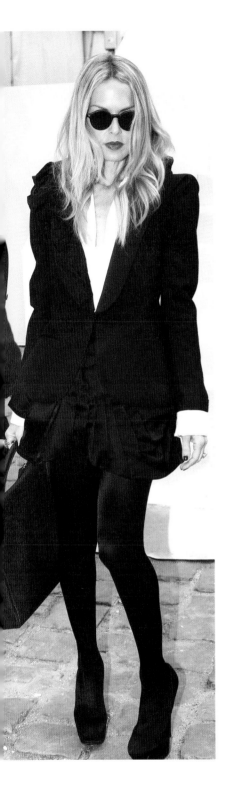

MAX OUT: Do not fear the maxi dress. I swear, it works for everyone. If you're petite, wear it with heels (and be sure the hemline still touches the floor) or opt for one that is more fitted with less volume.

BETWEEN THE LINES: Contrary to what people say, horizontal stripes do not always add bulk. I find that skinnier stripes—such as the ones on a French sailor sweater—are the most flattering. Trust me: Stripes actually make you look taller. Also, a racer stripe on the side of a pair of pants tricks the eye and makes you look leaner by elongating the leg.

LEAN LIMBS: A bishop's sleeve, which is fitted from the shoulder to the elbow and then flares slightly, always looks elegant and leans out the upper arms.

NECKLINE KNOW-HOW: A choker worn just above the collarbone will make your neck appear longer. I swear by this one. Long necklaces—with a dress or separates—also extend the line of the body, so you look taller and slimmer overall.

GO NUDE: To create the illusion of longer legs, slip into a pair of nude platform wedges or pumps—the higher, the better. Be sure to match the shade to your skin tone—whether it's a true taupe or more of a dusky pale rose—so that the pumps appear to be an extension of your gams. Avoid T-straps, which bisect the line and shorten the leg.

WHITE HOT: I adore white all year round because it brightens the skin. It makes you look fresh and stand out in a sea of black. Experiment with different shades to find what complements your complexion. Stark snow white can wash out someone fair, but works best for darker skin tones. A silk white, winter white, or off-white—*blanc cassé* in French—could be much more flattering for you.

KICK OFF: Dark denim is *always* more slimming than a lighter wash. A pair of midrise jeans with a kick or flare below the knee—whether it is a wide-leg or a boot-cut style—is elongating for everyone, I promise you. I love skinny jeans, but the reality is they are not universally flattering; tall, boyish figures fare best in the silhouette.

MY FASHION UNIFORM

The idea of a uniform may sound drab to you, but it's actually the best-kept secret of every stylish woman. If there's one thing I learned as a stylist, it's that no one—not even movie stars with outrageous bodies—wakes up super excited to get dressed every single morning. Even some of the most gorgeous actresses have issues with their bodies. Besides, some days you just feel exhausted or uninspired. Maybe you danced until 3:00 a.m. Maybe your precious toddler crawled into your bed and said, "Wake up, Mommy!" in the middle of the night.

> "WHETHER YOU'RE A WORKING WOMAN, A FULL-TIME STUDENT, OR A NEW MOM, YOU SHOULDN'T COMPROMISE YOUR STYLE. FOR SURE, FUNCTIONAL CAN BE FASHIONABLE."

I have a few different uniforms, depending upon where I am working and whom I will see on any given day. On a usual day in Los Angeles, my go-to look is basically a pair of wide-leg or bell-bottom jeans worn with a T-shirt, tunic, or tank and a statement jacket. For footwear, it's usually platform wedges that allow me to move around fast and comfortably. I definitely have a practical sensibility, but still always aim to look chic. Whether you're a working woman, a full-time student, or a new mom, you shouldn't compromise your style. For sure, functional can be fashionable. Before I even enter my closet in the morning, I ask myself three questions.

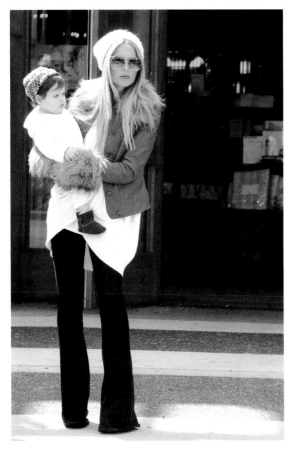
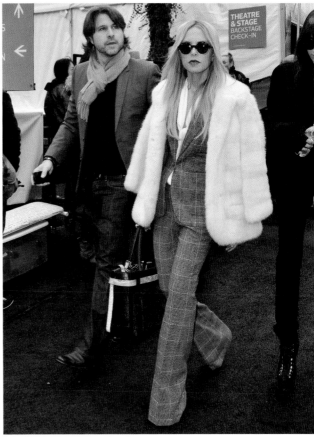

Left: A typical NYC "uniform."
Right: A typical LA "uniform."

WHAT'S ON MY SCHEDULE? First, I muse on my entire day—from tasks to appointments—and consider which clothes will carry me through every hour. If I know I will be running from one meeting to another or standing all day at a fitting, I opt for outfits that move with me. No fussy silk blouses or heavy accessories. You might see me in a maxi skirt with a soft tee and a knit duster.

WHO AM I SEEING TODAY? Am I tweaking a collection all day in the showroom with my team? My outfit can be stripped down and easy: high-waisted denim with a cashmere sweater and heels. But if clients are coming into the office or I'm styling an actress for an event, I add a structured jacket with a lot of hardware. It's smart to save those super-chic accents for days when you really need them.

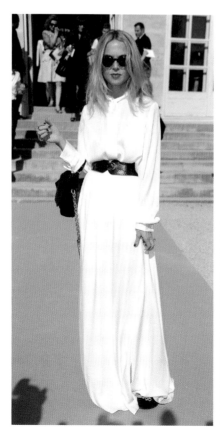 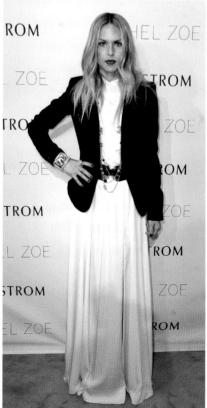

HOW LONG IS MY DAY? It's very rare that my working day ends at sunset. I always make time to run home to feed Skyler and put him down to sleep before I head back out for a dinner or fashion event. Still, I get dressed in the morning with my evening agenda in mind. You might dash to drinks, a business dinner, or a date right from work. To make that transition from office to after-hours as seamless as possible, wear an outfit that transforms easily. A simple black jumpsuit, for instance, gets an upgrade with a fur vest, higher heels, and a few gold cuffs. And don't forget to add a smoky eye or a red lip.

Of course, I always infuse my day-to-day look with a little glamour. My fashion talisman is a pair of black tuxedo pants. I swear, they are magic when it comes to amping up a simple outfit. My preference is a pair in a good crepe or georgette that won't wrinkle during the day and I always insist on a little stretch so that they give when I'm dashing around. A pair of great dark jeans that look crisp and clean can always work for me, too. Once you nail your uniform, it's easy to shop for chic variations on it.

WHEN IN DOUBT, EVOLVE

Yes, finding a signature look is key. But never straying from that look or updating it will land you in a rut. Your style is a lot like any long-term relationship. If you don't shake things up once in a while and experiment, boredom sneaks in. If I look at pictures of myself over the past decade, I can see a decided shift in my style.

At any given moment five or so years ago, you would have found me wafting around in an ethereal floor-length caftan with huge sunnies, eighteen necklaces, and strappy brown sandals—even in the middle of January. I was going for this South of France vibe all year round. Maybe I took living in L.A. too literally. Nowadays, my style is a lot less bohemian and slightly more practical—I like to think that it's more refined and polished. For inspiration now, I look to street style in cities like Paris and London instead of far-flung beaches. I can think of six great reasons to reevaluate your closet.

"YOUR STYLE IS A LOT LIKE ANY LONG-TERM RELATIONSHIP. IF YOU DON'T SHAKE THINGS UP ONCE IN A WHILE AND EXPERIMENT, BOREDOM SNEAKS IN."

Left: In a vintage
Missoni caftan, 2008.
Right: In a maternity
look.

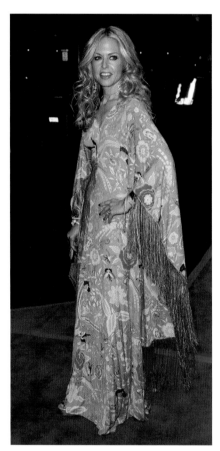
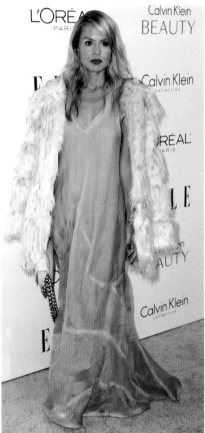

HAVING A CHILD: I can't even begin to list the many wonderful ways motherhood has changed my life, but I will say that my clothes are no longer as precious. Most outfits must be more durable and able to withstand tugs from tiny hands and sticky fingerprint smears. I choose soft cottons and crepe wools over delicate fabrics such as silk chiffon or crochet knits. Maybe that's why I wear so much black now, too!

FALLING IN OR OUT OF LOVE: Clearly, a life pivot like going solo after a long-term relationship calls for a fresh eye on your wardrobe. Maybe it's time to reinvent your look—even dress up a little more. Similarly, a new romance—or a sudden crush—is a great excuse to take stock of your sartorial staples or try something new.

CAREER MOVE: When I added fashion designer to my résumé, I needed to revamp my look for meetings with conservative investors and buttoned-up buyers. My urban boho style begged for more architecture and edge with an infusion of sophisticated and tailored pieces. I added structured bags to my accessories and swapped teetering sandals for more empowered platform pumps and ankle boots. The metamorphosis didn't just alter my appearance, though. With my new career—and a staff of thirty executives, editors, stylists, and assistants to oversee—I needed pieces that made me feel more effectual and authoritative.

SCALE FLUCTUATION: Obviously, pregnancy calls for roomier clothes. For me, maternity wear consisted mostly of bubble dresses, leggings, long caftans, and lots of scarves to deflect the focus from my expanding waist.

Still, any time you gain or lose more than ten or fifteen pounds, you should try on your clothes and reassess the fit. A tailor can nip in or let out a seam if you go down or up a size. If it requires more than a quick fix, decide if you plan to stay at this new weight and shop accordingly. Wearing clothes that constrict will only gnaw at your self-esteem, and the same goes for garments that are now too large and barely skim your figure.

NEW HOME: A major move calls for a wardrobe check. When I first moved from Manhattan to Los Angeles, my all-black staples from power suits to body-con dresses suddenly felt severe and forced. On the West Coast, effortless chic rules. No one wears tights or conservative black pumps or even pleats. I have seen film executives in flip-flops! Back in New York and other East Coast cities, breezing into a boardroom in an ikat silk maxi dress and gold gladiator sandals will get you demoted. So if you relocate from a small town to a city or to a whole new time zone, be sure to take note of the style of your new locale. You don't have to conform, but you might find some surprising and flattering new additions to your look if you're open to adapting. Of course, a dramatic climate change requires new staples.

MILESTONE BIRTHDAY: Whether you're turning twenty-five or forty, a significant birthday is an ideal time to scrutinize your inventory. First of all, you can figure out what you want to splurge on and think of it as a gift to yourself. Do you need a leopard-print belt or a pair of riding boots? Treat yourself. Second, there's a chance that you have outgrown—both figuratively and literally—a few items. Ten years ago, I wore tailored shorts, which I no longer do. That's not to say that you should toss your short skirts or shorts when you say hello to forty as a rule. It's more of a personal comfort level and yes, a matter of taste. At forty, it may be time to retire the midriff-baring tops and cut-off denim shorts. But then again, some women still manage to pull it off, so maybe not. A milestone is a good time to reassess, nonetheless.

VINTAGE: HUNTING AND GATHERING

Without a doubt, my love for vintage has formed the foundation of my signature style. Even as a teenager, I had no interest in wearing the latest trend or designer du jour. If it was cool to wear what everyone else wore, I bypassed cool. While my friends in New Jersey bought Benetton sweaters and Guess jeans, I browsed the flea market stands in Soho for mod shifts and major costume jewelry.

One reason for collecting vintage is simply that in most cases, no one else will have it. When I first started styling, I knew that adding vintage accessories and pieces into my clients' red-carpet looks would make them stand out. But wearing a midcentury modern big brass cuff or a vintage biker jacket also relays this instinctive sense of style. It shows that you can breeze into a retro boutique or thrift shop or estate sale and strike gold (sometimes literally).

When I was younger, buying vintage was also a way to access fantastic pieces on a meager budget. Some of my favorite looks cost under fifty dollars. I can still recall this architectural military jacket I found in a thrift shop that I wore to death. There was a leather bomber jacket, too. (Clearly, my jacket fetish started early on.) But my biggest vintage coup back in the day was a seventies Gucci coat with original horse-bit accents. It's still hanging in my closet and looks as glamourous today as it did twenty-five years ago.

It's easy to go crazy and buy everything chic in sight. Trust me, I know. These days, I seek out only seminal designer pieces that bear a stamp or label. (That was Rodger's advice after watching me take over every single inch of closet space in our home.) My friend William Banks-Blaney in London has an insane vintage boutique and he drops me a line if he gets in a breathtaking Dior cocktail dress, a YSL piece from one of his most famous collections, or an amazing Courrèges jacket. Over the years, I have willed myself to think twice, even three times, before I purchase yet another caftan or cocktail ring. In Chapter 3, my mom, Leslie, will share her tried-and-true tips on shopping vintage, but here's what goes through my head before I get to the register.

DOES IT FIT? A great but ill-fitting piece might be inexpensive, but I always consider the cost of tailoring, too. Reconstructing a dress or jacket can add up, so I never buy anything that will cost as much as its price tag to tailor to my measurements. In essence, ask yourself, "Is it more work than it's worth?"

IS IT IN GOOD CONDITION? I recommend that you avoid damaged pieces—especially if they date back to the pre-fifties, when fabrics were manufactured differently. A small tear is an easy fix for a tailor; obvious stains or elbows that have frayed or thinned require costly cosmetic surgery—and even then, they may never look exactly right.

WILL IT UPDATE? Some vintage pieces can easily be modernized with the addition of a contemporary top, jacket, or shoes. But certain looks—like thick polyester jackets from the seventies or heavy brocade column dresses—will always look costumey and should be avoided.

IS IT REALLY AN INVESTMENT? I have heard many stories of fake designer labels being sewn into marginal designs. If you're looking to splurge on a piece for its heritage, be sure that the label matches the time period—e.g., YSL updates its label every decade—and that the vintage seller has a stellar reputation. Websites such as VintageFashionGuild.com offer authentication resources like a directory of designer labels such as Loris Azzaro and Gilbert Adrian for cross-reference. I also love 1stdibs.com and RessurectionVintage.com, because they give you a little history about a particular piece and you know everything is authentic.

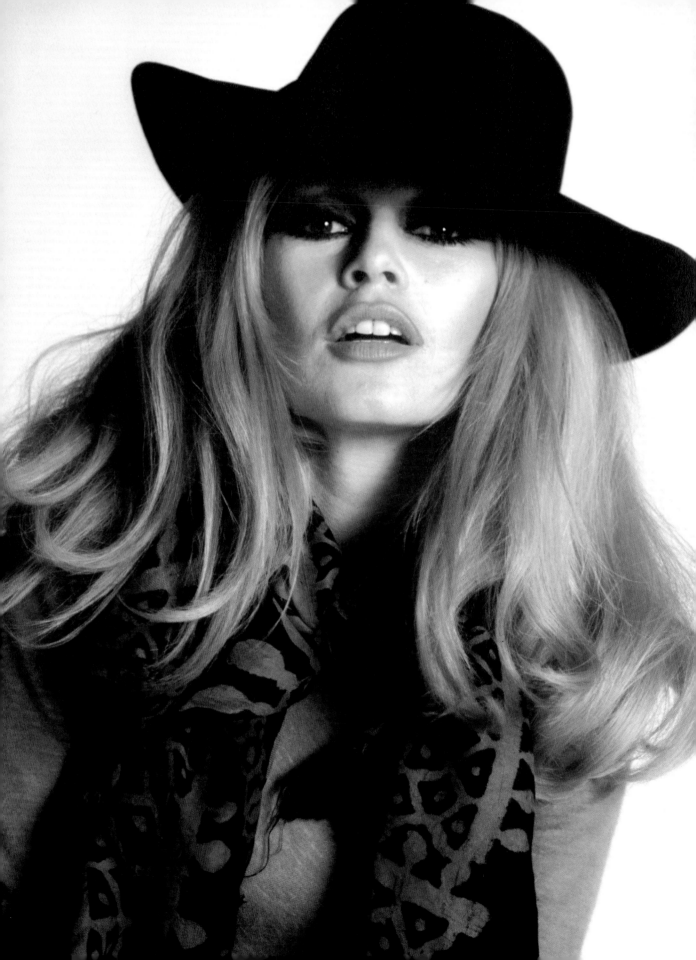

Brigitte Bardot

MY STYLE ICONS

It's no surprise that I look to the past for style cues. As I've said, my own aesthetic is anchored in a carefree elegance that reigned in fashion during the sixties and seventies. When I'm musing on my next collection or dressing a client for the red carpet, I always think about the amazingly stylish women who constantly influence me. Each of these icons inspires me in a completely different way, whether it's to play up the sexy appeal of androgyny or to steer more toward an ethereal romanticism. Meet my top ten women of style and enjoy some tips on how you can emulate their glamour with a few key pieces.

THE EVERYDAY BOMBSHELL: BRIGITTE BARDOT
"Every age can be enchanting, provided you live within it."

If only we all woke up looking like my absolute idol. Somehow, Bardot—with her sensually tangled hair and dramatic cat-eye makeup—always nailed effortless glamour. It was as though she had just stepped out of a Mercedes convertible after doing her hair and makeup at seventy-five miles per hour. Even wearing a simple sundress with casual sandals around the South of France, she managed to look extremely sexy without ever looking cheap.

Closet must-haves: An off-the-shoulder sundress, striped bateau sweater, and ballet flats. Accent the look with a thick headband and delicate gold chains.

THE SCENE QUEEN: BIANCA JAGGER

"I don't want to wear what every other woman wears. I won't be dictated to."

Leave it to the Studio 54 staple and Mick Jagger's former muse to wink at masculinity and look even more feminine for it. Jagger wore a custom white Yves Saint Laurent skirt suit to her 1971 Saint-Tropez wedding, and had a penchant for strong lines and tailored silhouettes. But she knew to dabble heavily in Halston's buttery, fluid sheaths whenever she hit the dance floor. She not only defines glamour and sexiness, but disco, too. I reference her often when I'm styling or getting dressed for a night out.

Closet must-haves: A tailored slim-cut suit to wear with pumps and a lace camisole. One vintage seventies disco dress, preferably sequined or threaded with gold Lurex. A long pendant necklace and an envelope clutch make great finishing touches.

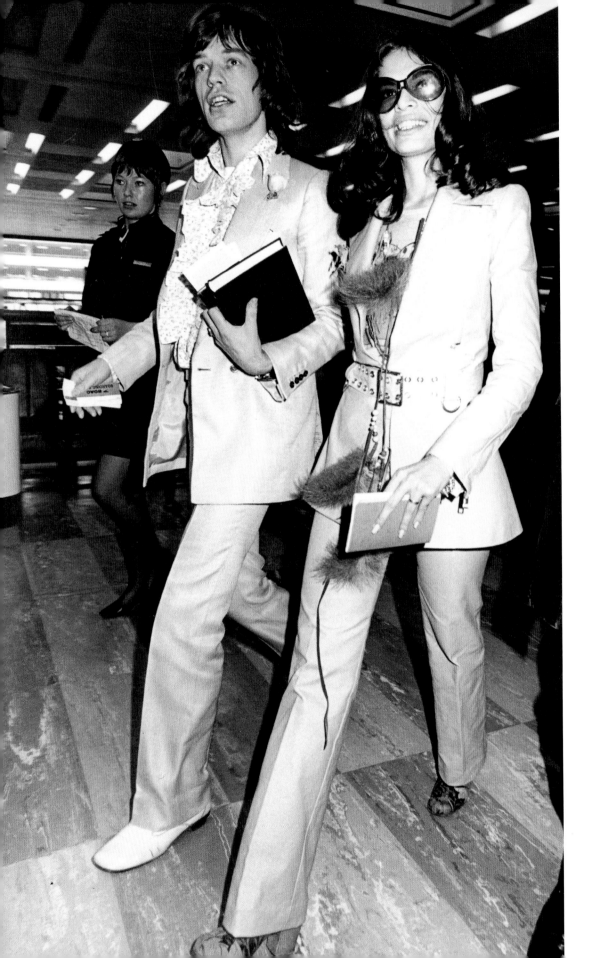

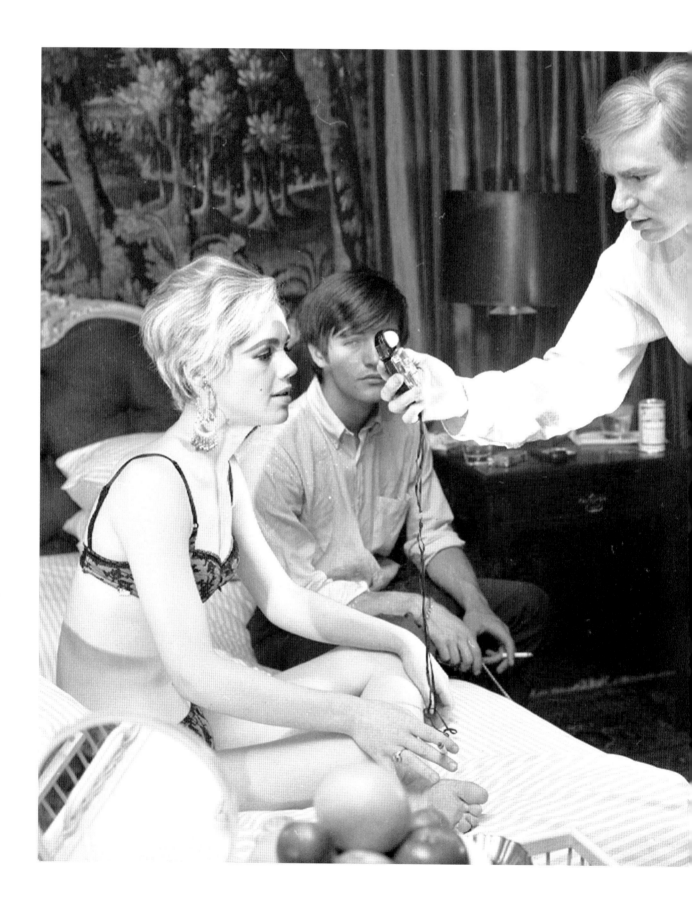

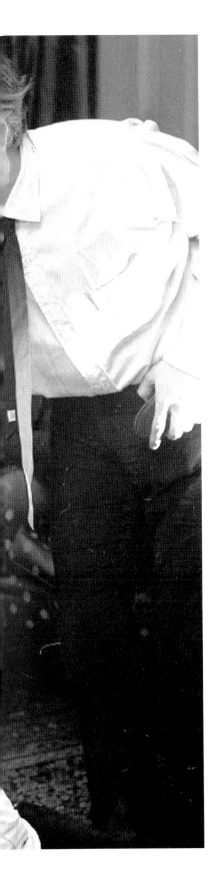

THE MIDCENTURY MOD WAIF: EDIE SEDGWICK

"It's not that I'm rebelling. It's that I'm just trying to find another way."

I never get tired of staring at pictures of the socialite whom *Vogue* once called a "youthquaker." With her pale lips, outrageous lashes, and striped blond pixie hair, she defined that whole era of linear sixties mod. I particularly love that she trotted around New York in a black leotard, tights, and a T-shirt because she practiced ballet twice a day—and that this simple look became an "it girl" costume. It's a perfect example of how a signature style can identify you and become a classic.

Closet must-haves: Opaque black tights with a metallic minidress and a mod leopard print coat. Add tassel earrings and lots of Lucite cuffs as points of interest, too.

Edie Sedgwick on set with Andy Warhol

THE CHIC PREP: ALI MACGRAW

"Looking at beautiful things is what makes me the happiest."

With that sleek curtain of shiny black hair and strong, striking features, this classic beauty epitomized the best of Ivy League style. Sure, her role in *Love Story* created a camel hair craze, but her bohemian tomboy look offscreen is worthy of a once-over, too. Her preppy wardrobe staples included knit caps, sleek trousers, and peasant blouses. MacGraw's early style always reminds me of modern-day Ralph Lauren. She really mastered androgyny, but added her own feminine flair with turbans and velvet chokers. I love the photos of her pre-actress days as a model and an assistant to Diana Vreeland at *Vogue*.

Closet must-haves: A long fitted sweater vest and a well-worn pair of brown equestrian boots. Add a knit cloche and chunky Navajo jewelry as accessories.

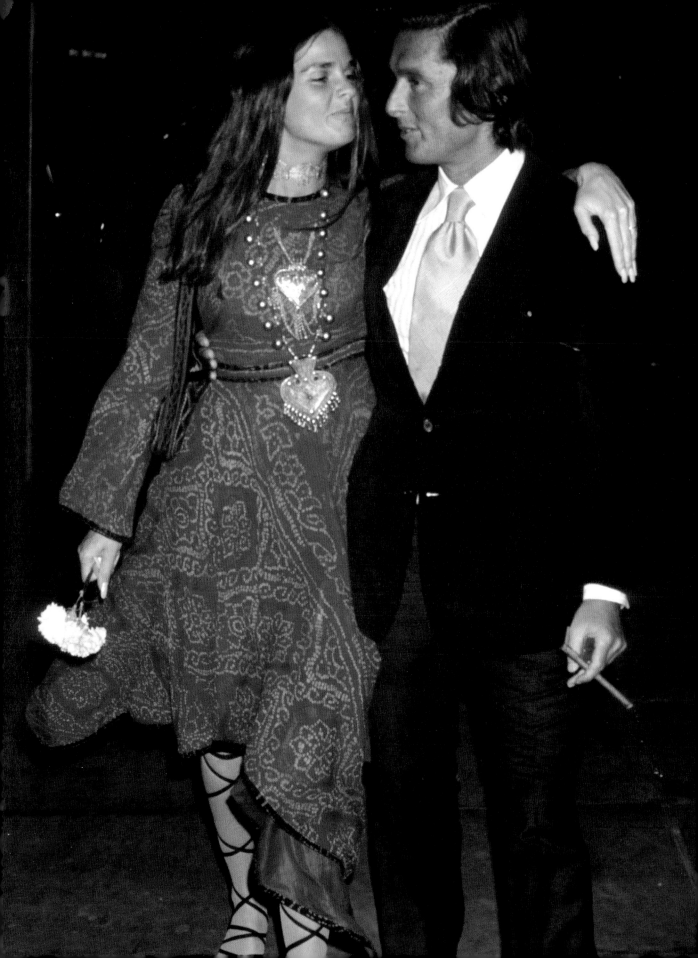

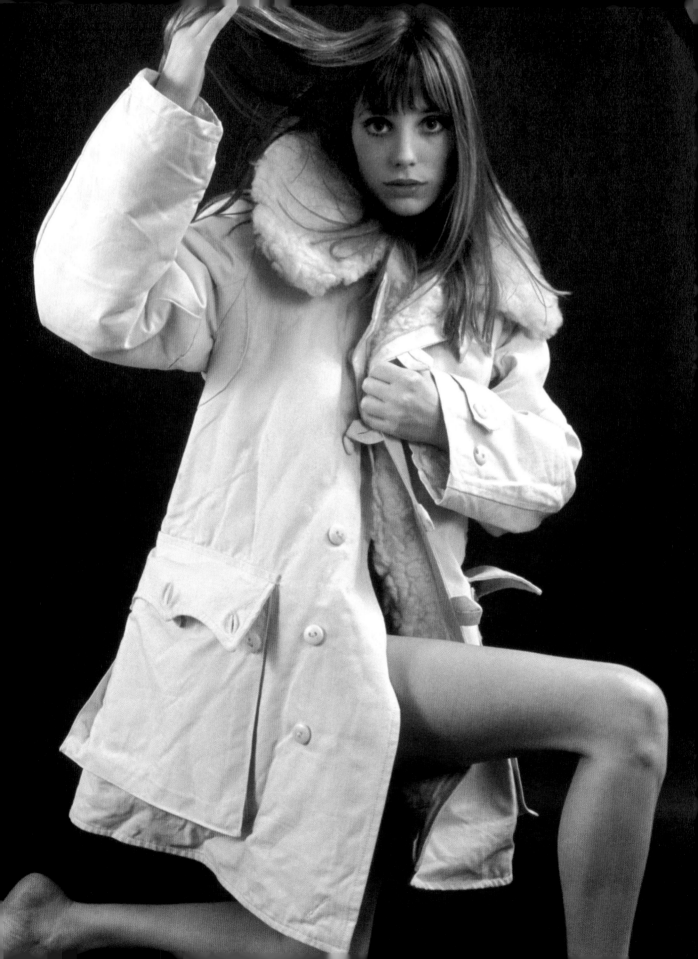

Jane Birkin

THE FRENCH CHANTEUSE: JANE BIRKIN

"Keep smiling. It takes ten years off!"

Never mind her huge caramel eyes and those long blunt bangs, this gorgeous woman had an innate sense of personal style that everyone still tries to emulate. It was schoolgirl poet in her short, sweet dresses mixed with nonchalant street chic with her high-waisted denim and peacoats. She's one of my biggest influences when I design. In fact, I think every fashion designer has at least one Jane Birkin moment. She had this habit of never matching and yet her outfits always came together so perfectly. Hermès named what's become their most iconic bag after her—what could be cooler than that?

Closet must-haves: A sixties-style A-line shift, cropped velvet pants, and a pair of Parisian-chic leather ankle boots. Look for a long vintage pendant necklace and slender gold bangles to complete the look.

THE FOLK HEROINE: MARIANNE FAITHFULL

"I wear Chanel. It doesn't go in and out of fashion at all."

There is so much soul to this woman's look, whether she's outfitted in a peasant dress and floppy hat or a miniskirt and silver Mary Janes. Faithfull battled a lot of demons in her early life and her style reflected her struggles and identities—from the happy hippie songbird to the raw, exposed rocker chick. You can see both those sides in her shaggy protective bangs, leather frocks, and high boots. She screams retro rock-and-roll London to me and I can't get enough of that.

Closet must-haves: A lace minidress, flat black ankle boots, and a floral print blazer. Accessorize with a distressed leather backpack and a floppy felt fedora.

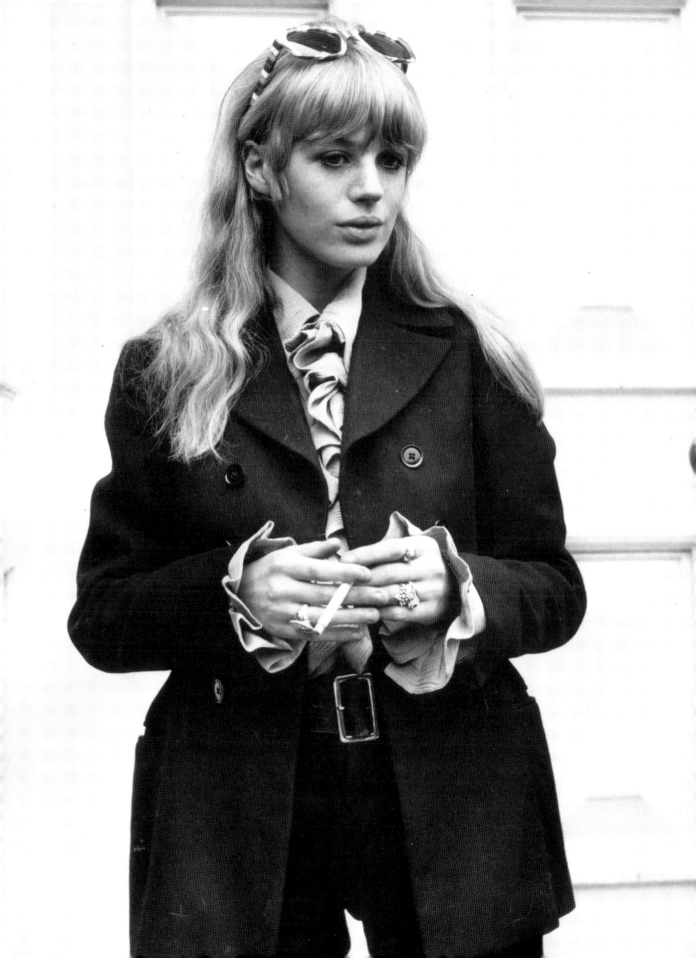

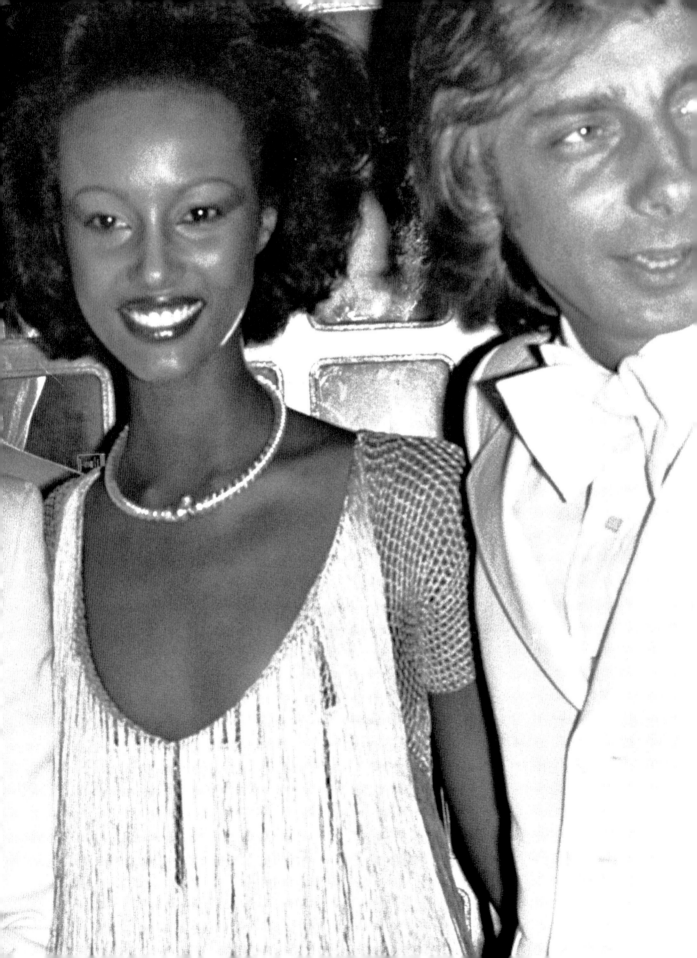

THE THINKING WOMAN'S SUPERMODEL: IMAN

"I believe in glamour. I am in favor of a little vanity. Looking good is a commitment to yourself and to others."

Iman and I first bonded over our shared obsession with the disco era and that decade's unabashed celebration of chic. No one rocks a metallic jumpsuit like this multitalented woman, I swear to you. When she wore a maxi skirt and blouse from my resort collection to accept a prestigious award in Beverly Hills in 2011, I nearly melted. Like me, Iman is obsessed with caftans and relies on statement accessories like bold jewelry and knockout shoes to complete her look. But it's her generous spirit and the way in which she carries herself that comes to mind when I look to her for inspiration. She's invincible—the strongest woman I know.

Closet must-haves: A velvet suit with flared pants and fitted jacket and a leather pencil skirt. A chain belt and a graphic choker are signature Iman accents, too.

THE SCREEN SIREN: SOPHIA LOREN

"Sex appeal is fifty percent what you've got and fifty percent what people think you've got."

Was there ever a time that this Italian superstar did not look drop-dead glamourous? I once saw her outside a Golden Globes party at the Beverly Hilton in Los Angeles, walked right up to her, and said, "I never, ever do this, but I have to say that you are AMAZING!" She smiled and replied in her silky Italian accent, "Thaaaank you so much." Loren, with her curves and exotic beauty, has sensuality and elegance down to a science. She wears a flouncy floral frock like it's a bandage dress and always manages to make cleavage a classy accessory in deep scoop necks and plunging V-necks.

Closet must-haves: A sleeveless dress with a flared skirt and fitted bodice. Of course, a few pieces of classic lingerie like satin tap pants and a tulle and lace corset. You can't go wrong with an oversized black straw sun hat and classic nude stiletto pumps as well.

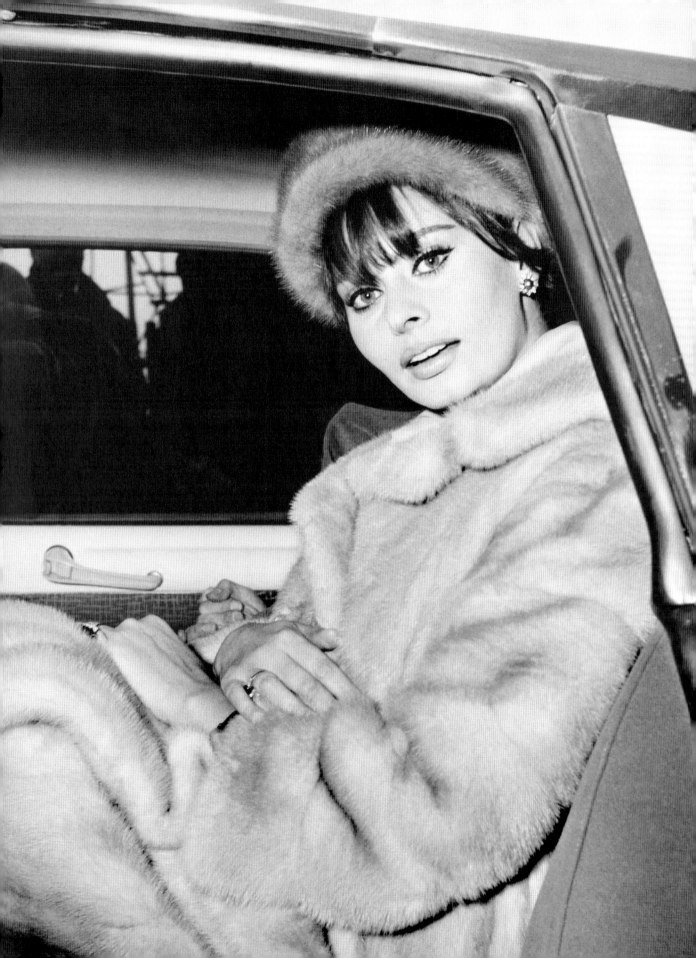

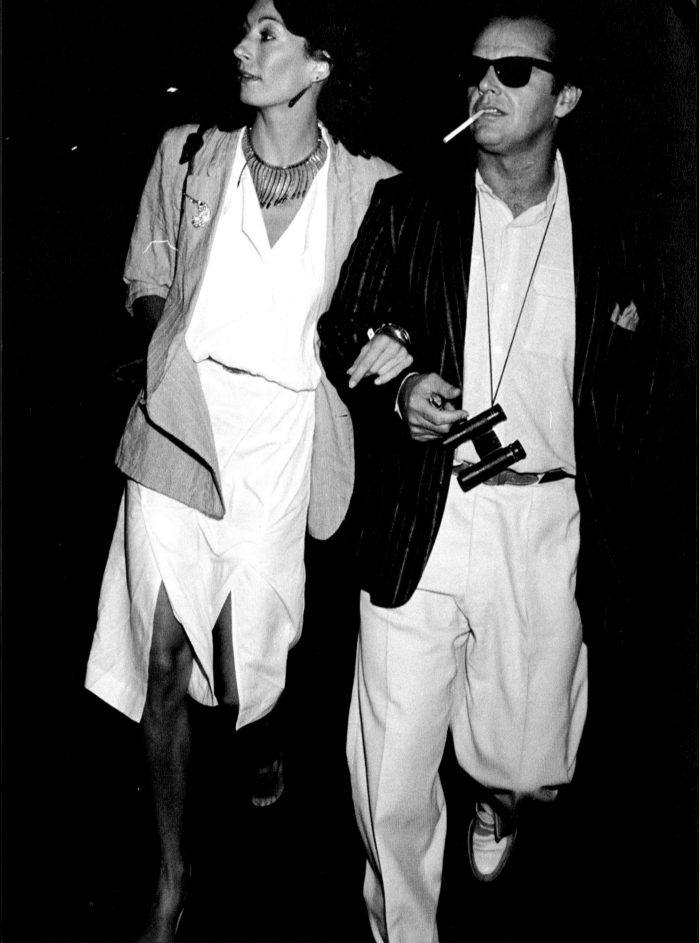

Anjelica Huston with Jack Nicholson

THE DESIGNER MUSE: ANJELICA HUSTON

"Nothing I buy ever looks new, because I have my look down and it's classic."

Models with perfect symmetrical faces couldn't compete with Huston and her bold Cubist features. I love that she highlighted her face as if it were a canvas by wearing her long raven hair in a sleek chignon. Back then, she stood out amid the blond-haired and blue-eyed models, and inspired women who didn't fit the all-American ideal of beauty. Her Irish roots showed in the way she wore tweed separates as eveningwear, and Huston never met a fitted blazer she didn't like. She was a muse and model for both Halston and Valentino in the sixties and seventies—enough said. I also named a pair of high-waisted wide-leg trousers after her in my first collection.

Closet must-haves: A black crepe jumpsuit with a deep V-neck that shows off your clavicle and a one-shoulder party dress. Vintage geometric scarves, a sleek structured bag, and don't-mess-with-me sculptural cuffs all make perfect add-ons.

THE POWER VIXEN: DIANE VON FURSTENBERG

"Your clothes are your friends. Be the woman you want to be."

Let me just say that this woman is the epitome of everything I strive to be—she's a personal hero for so many reasons. Beyond her unique beauty and dynamic sense of style, she exudes this strength and confidence that are just so captivating. She wears everything—from a sequined gown to denim and a tunic—with such authority and ease. If you look at pictures throughout her career, you can see that she has never feared splashy prints and color. Her outfits, even now, always skim her curves and suggest (rather than announce) her sexuality. She's extraordinary in that she's an icon to so many generations of women, even inspiring today's younger set.

Closet must-haves: A wrap dress, of course, long printed dresses, and a sleek fitted blazer that you can push up at the arms. An animal-print cashmere scarf and a clutch with bold hardware work perfectly as accents.

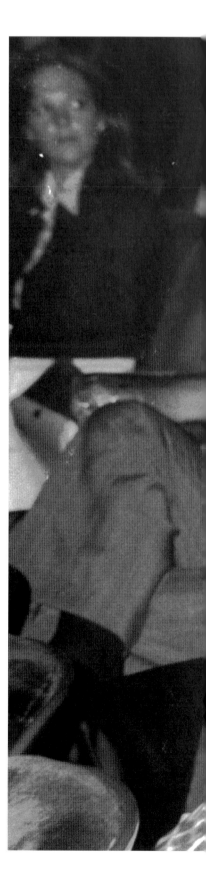

Diane von Furstenberg

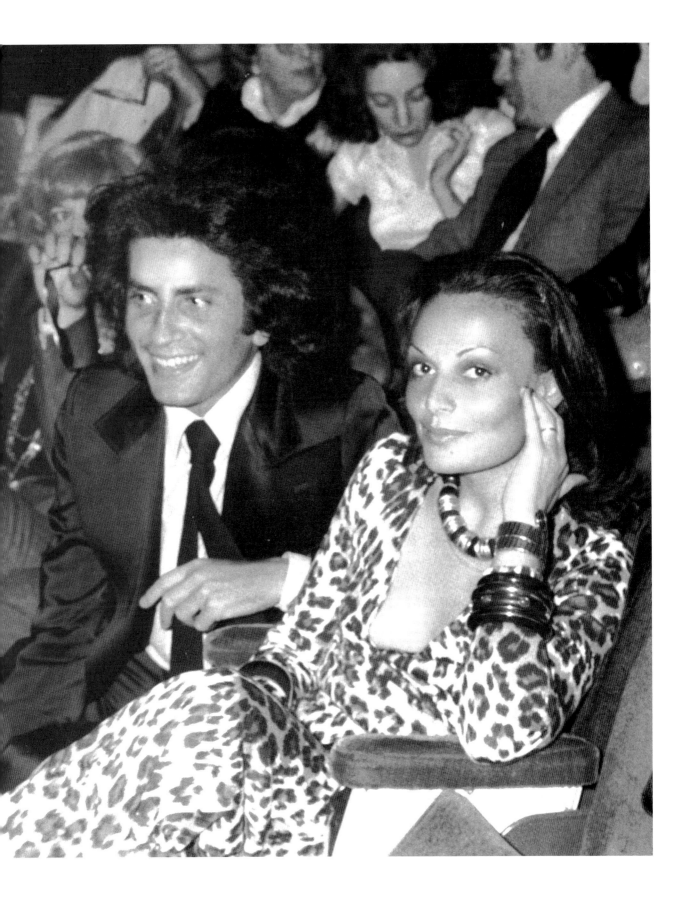

CAMERA READY

The red carpet terrifies me. I have been photographed many times at this point, but I would be lying if I said I feel at ease with flashbulbs in my face. That said, I try to follow the tips I pass along to my clients for nailing a photo op.

Bypass the shimmer and glitter. That dewy look we all love often reads as perspiration in a photo.

When posing, to avoid coming across as stiff and very pageantlike, just keep your arms relaxed at your sides to show off your outfit.

Berry lips with a blue undertone make teeth look whiter. Nude and magenta hues aren't as flattering.

Small prints have a tendency to strobe or blur in a photo, so go with a solid or a larger graphic print.

Play Mario Testino. I take pictures of my clients from every angle—the back, the front, the side, from above and below—before I send them off to face the paparazzi. You can check your makeup by taking a quick shot in natural light and then ask a friend to photograph you full-length as I do for my clients.

While a sleek chignon can be the most elegant of coifs, it can look severe in a photo because you can't see the actual bun. I always pull out a few wisps around the face to soften the style.

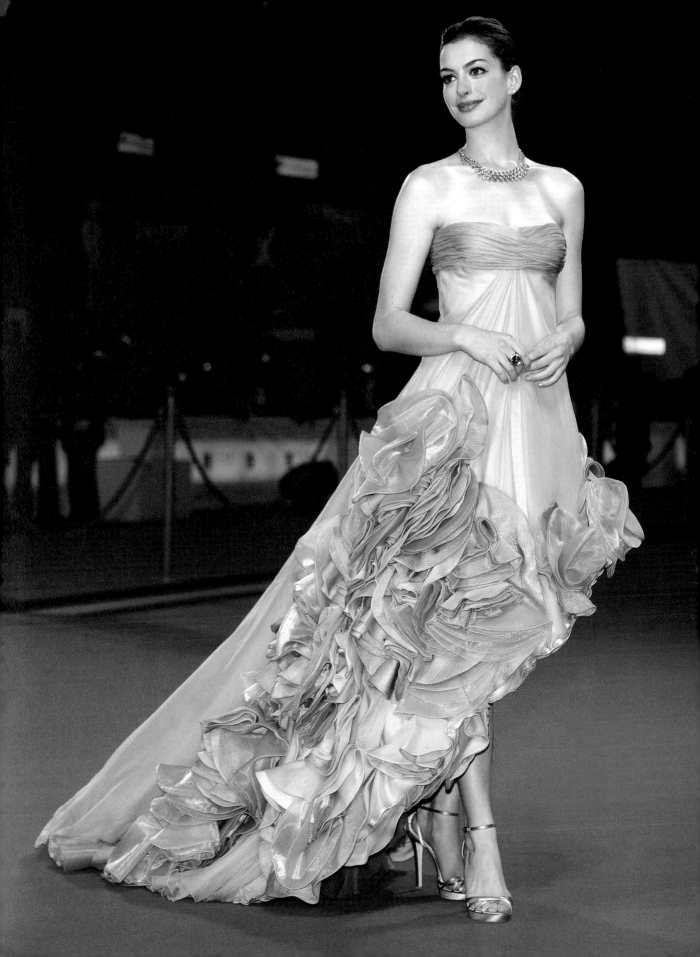

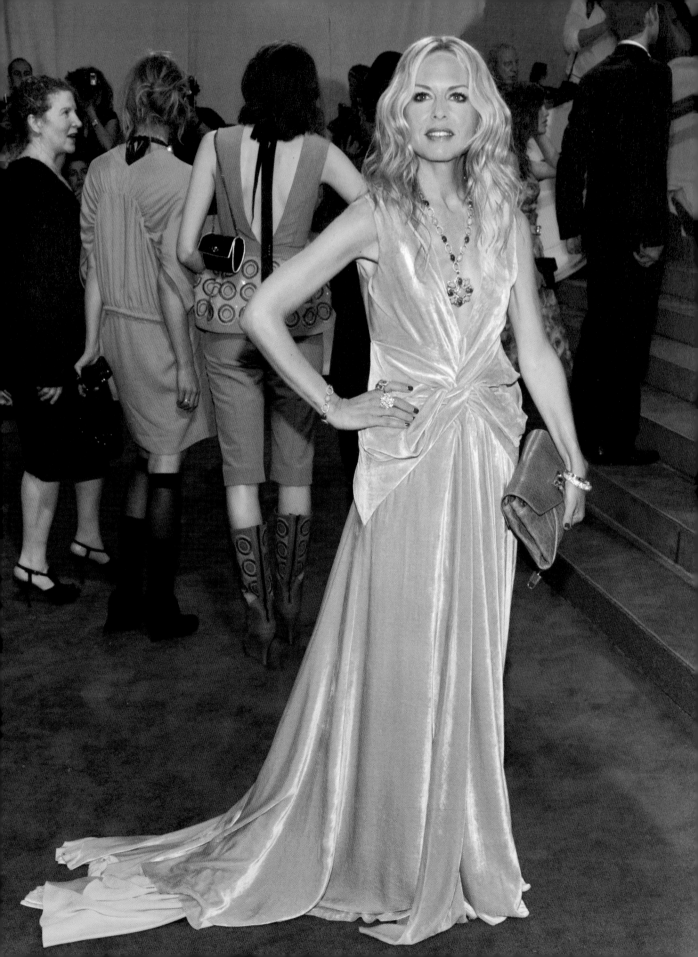

TAKE A FASHION LEAP

Once you have found your fashion comfort zone, take a risk. If you always wear long sleeves, I dare you to slip into a strapless dress. Think you loathe the color red? Stop by a makeup counter and experiment with a berry lip. When it comes to style, my mantra is: "Just try it once." That applies to my own daily wardrobe decisions as well as to my work as a designer and a stylist. I once wore a vibrant yellow velvet Marc Jacobs gown to the Met Gala.

> "ONCE YOU HAVE FOUND YOUR FASHION
> COMFORT ZONE, TAKE A RISK."

Yes, I had stepped out of my fashion comfort zone. But in the end, I felt really special wearing my friend's dress on such a major fashion night. It was definitely a "moment" for me.

When I first meet with an actress as a stylist, I always ask her if she's "highly allergic" to any colors and which silhouettes scare her. I sit and I nod—like a therapist—and then I start to plot her first big fashion risk. My client Jennifer Garner once told me that she would never wear a one-shoulder dress. Guess what? The vintage one-shoulder tangerine Valentino gown she wore for the Oscars in 2004 still stands as one of her favorite looks to date. Anne Hathaway, another longtime client and dear friend, told me when we first met that like me, she would not wear yellow. You know where this story is going, right? And the list goes on and on.

> "WHEN IT COMES TO STYLE,
> MY MANTRA IS: 'JUST TRY IT ONCE.'"

Fashion should be thrilling and unpredictable and fun. All my icons have become forever memorable because they loved to express themselves through their style. If you're cultivating your signature look, enjoy every ounce of the experimentation. Laugh at your reflection when you try on something unflattering. Squeal a little if a dress or a pair of jeans makes you look utterly fantastic. And be sure to take a risk every now and again. Go ahead, I dare you.

CHAPTER 3

DETAIL ORIENTED

Black patent ankle boots or nude platform pumps? A bold enamel pendant necklace or a pair of geometric cuffs? In my opinion, an outfit is only half complete without accessories. When I get dressed in the morning, I think about all the possibilities—from a hat to the necklace to the shoes—as I decide on a look. Sometimes, I like to start backward and select my jewelry first. Then, I might choose a simple black sheath or a crisp white button-down with flared trousers as the perfect canvas for a bold piece. It's no wonder I have been known to say "I dream in jewelry." Leaving the house without accessories would feel to me like walking out the door naked.

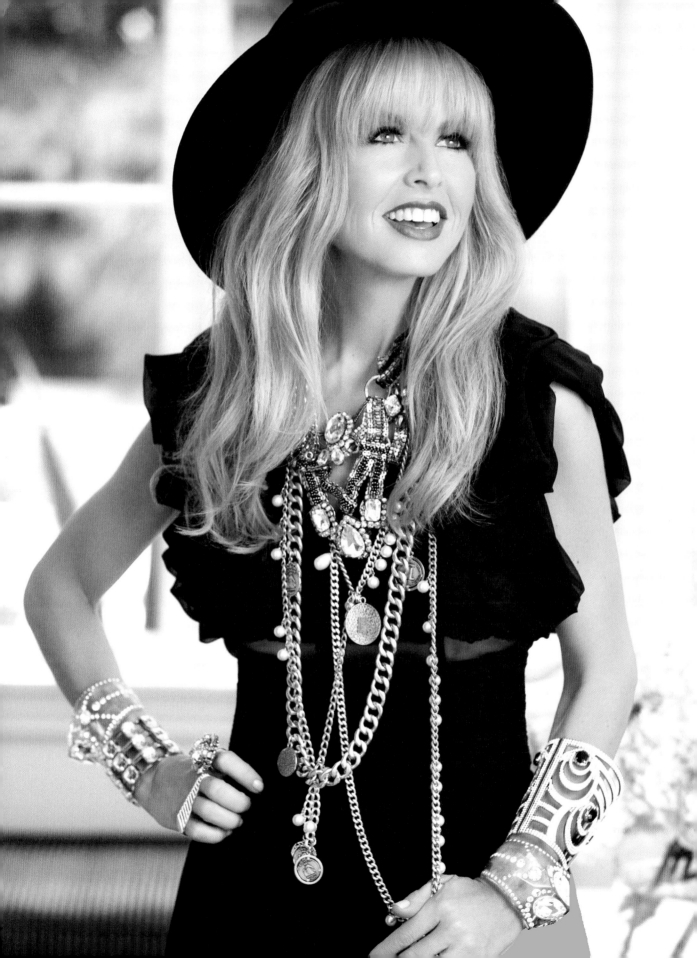

As I mentioned earlier, my mother always had a fabulous arsenal of accessories. If you look at pictures of her from when she was in her twenties and thirties, she is consistently decked out in oversized sunnies and huge necklaces. As a little girl, I swear that I could practically cover my whole body in all her bold chokers, pendants, strands of beads, cuffs, and cocktail rings. I never liked dainty pieces either. When I was sixteen, I bought my first piece of collectible costume jewelry: a Chanel charm bracelet at a vintage boutique in Paris. It was a big deal, because I had saved up for the thick gold chain, with a dangling Eiffel Tower and rue Cambon. I can still recall how it felt on my wrist—it was very heavy!—and sparkled in the sunlight. After that, I spent time saving up for a Louis Vuitton monogram purse. My parents thought I was crazy to splurge on a designer bag, but I already knew then that a chic, timeless investment like that would transform my day-to-day look.

"I SEE BOLD ACCESSORIES AS A WOMAN'S ARMOR."

Since then, my taste in accessories has undergone plenty of incarnations. My preteen obsession with everything gold led me to pile on stars, hearts, and lots of other flashy charms. During the early eighties, I had a thing for fingerless lace gloves, headbands, and white Ray-Bans. Later on in my college years, I went through a tribal phase of wearing chunky, Navajo-inspired jewelry, lots of turquoise and coral rings, and heavy silver necklaces. But no matter my style at any given time, I never, ever thought small. In the past decade or so, I have returned to my roots. I adore gold, especially chains with heft and oversized pendants. You can upgrade any look, from a bathing suit to a classic black turtleneck, with oversized accents of rich, lustrous gold.

I see bold accessories as a woman's armor. Look at Wonder Woman, with her chic gold cuffs, tiara, and those amazing red go-go boots. Cleopatra, known for her opulent accessories, adorned her headdresses with gold cobras and precious scarabs to convince all of Egypt she was a divine goddess. I could stare at pictures of Elizabeth Taylor from the 1963 film *Cleopatra*—not to mention, in general—all day for inspiration. Great accessories have their own special powers for me, too. A cool fedora is always my go-to on a bad hair day. If I need to feel confident for a meeting, I wear my stunning Van Cleef & Arpels Jackie O cuff, a molten eighteen-karat gold piece from 1977 that the jeweler reissued in a limited edition. Its weight and shine alone instill me with extra courage.

In a necklace by Chanel

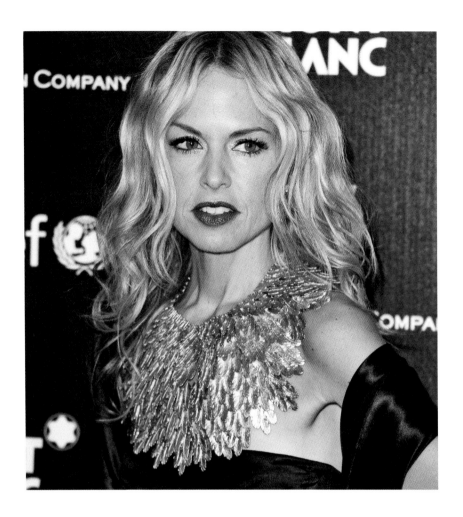

When I style an actress for the red carpet, the right jewelry or shoes can be the last piece of the puzzle. It might add a splash of color or a sense of texture—even a bit of avant-garde edge. The focus is almost always on the dress, but the right accessories always add a point of interest. In fact, they can even change the personality of a look. Here's an experiment: Take a little black dress out of your closet and model it in front of the mirror with different shoes, jewelry, and even a scarf or a hat. Add layered pearls and chains with lizard-skin sling-backs and you have the epitome of ladylike style. Change it up completely to nail downtown glamour with a chunky collar necklace, leather jacket, and ankle boots. Now you see why I sometimes pick my accessories first!

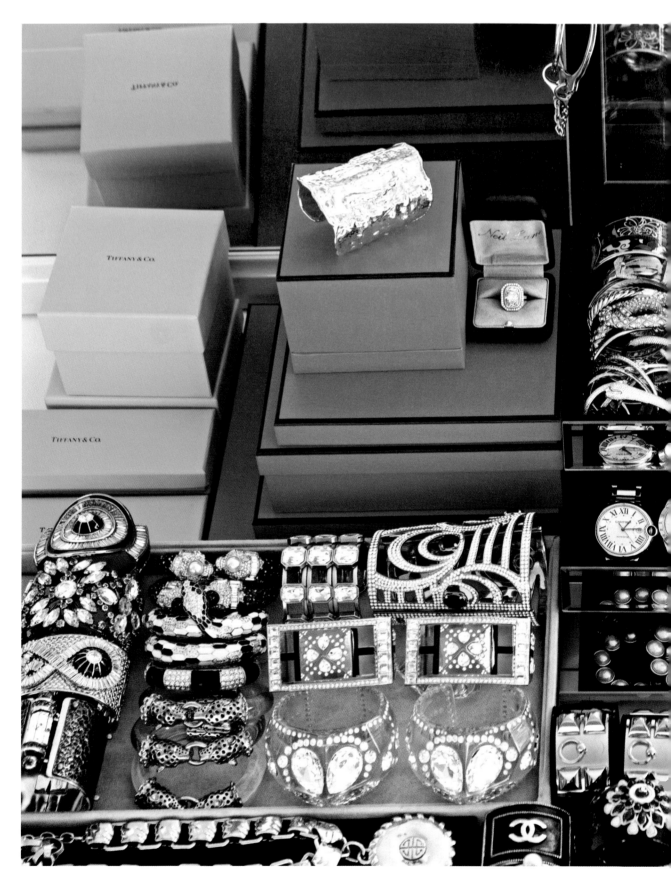

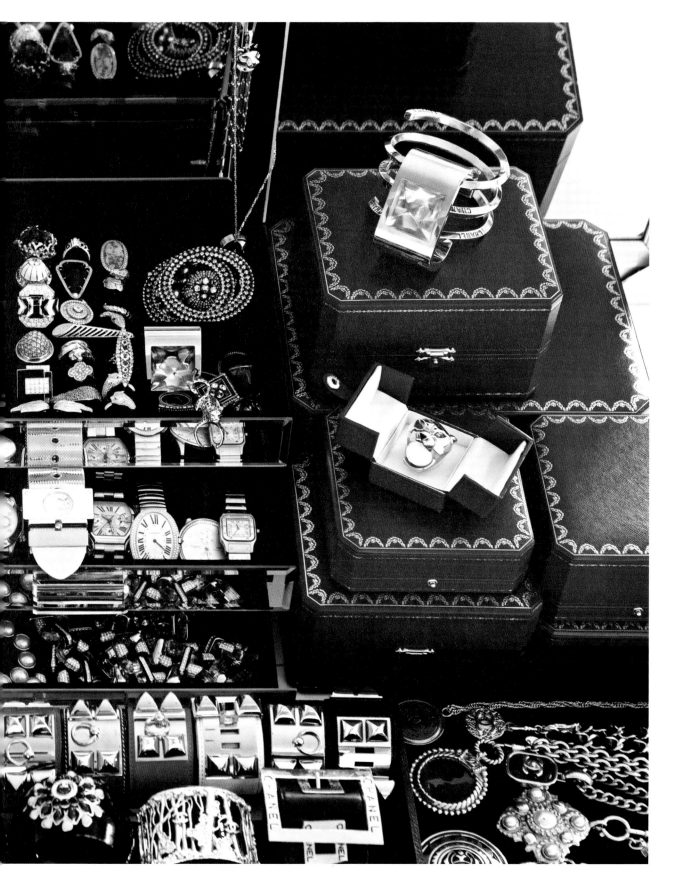

TRINKETS TO SUIT YOUR STYLE

Jewelry always tells a story. Rings, necklaces, and earrings often have some sentimental value and help us assume our style identities. One of my first prized pieces as a kid was a gold ring with little dangling hearts that announced my girly, flirtatious side. It was a gift for my bat mitzvah and I still have it in my jewelry box. When you start to collect jewelry or sit down to evaluate what you already own, think about your style. Do your pieces complement, even enhance, your fashion persona? Here are some style profiles to help guide your jewelry choices.

BOHEMIAN SPIRIT: You own a dozen peasant blouses, fringed purses, and never met a caftan you didn't adore. Your signature will probably be sizable gold hoops—think about the diameter of a silver dollar—that will stand out against your romantic waves. Long beaded chains or link necklaces that you can layer atop those ethnic prints are key. A few chunky turquoise, coral, or bone rings add some gypsy flair, too. But don't overdo it or you might look like you're wearing a costume!

"JEWELRY ALWAYS TELLS A STORY."

CHIC MINIMALIST: Clean simple silhouettes, streamlined proportions, and symmetry appeal to your love of only the bare essentials. The subtlety and architecture of a pair of pyramid studs will work perfectly when your hair is pin straight or pulled back into a tight chignon. An oversized men's watch, be it a Rolex or a Timex, and simple gold bands on your fingers also complement your pared-down style.

FASHION REBEL: Gwen Stefani is your style icon and your friends marvel at how only you can make leggings work with shorts in the office. A trio of cool huggies, studs, and spikes on your ear accent your unconventional street style. An oversized pendant necklace with geometric adornments, studded bangles, and a thick snake ring complete the look.

DRAMA QUEEN: You love metallic sequins for day and a one-shoulder dress is your go-to frock on any vacation—including a ski weekend in Aspen. Gold tassel drop earrings that sway with every head toss on a dance floor are essential. A few statement rings, a flashy gold choker with diamonds, or a group of oversized cuffs will get you noticed—in a good way.

UPTOWN GIRL: Cashmere cardigan in the closet? Check. Riding boots, too? Check. Headband? You're wearing it right now. Diamond studs are the classic, polished girl's best friend. I like them in baguettes, a princess cut, or even tiny flower configurations. A chic tank watch with an Hermès orange or rich cognac band looks great on your wrist, alongside a link bracelet with a monogrammed circle pendant.

Discovering your style narrative doesn't mean that you can't dabble in other profiles. I always say that every uptown girl should experiment, at least once, with an edgy downtown vibe. If you're a devout bohemian, take off a few bangles and pull that wild mane of hair into a sleek, straight ponytail. The most unique looks are actually a blend of a few contrasting elements.

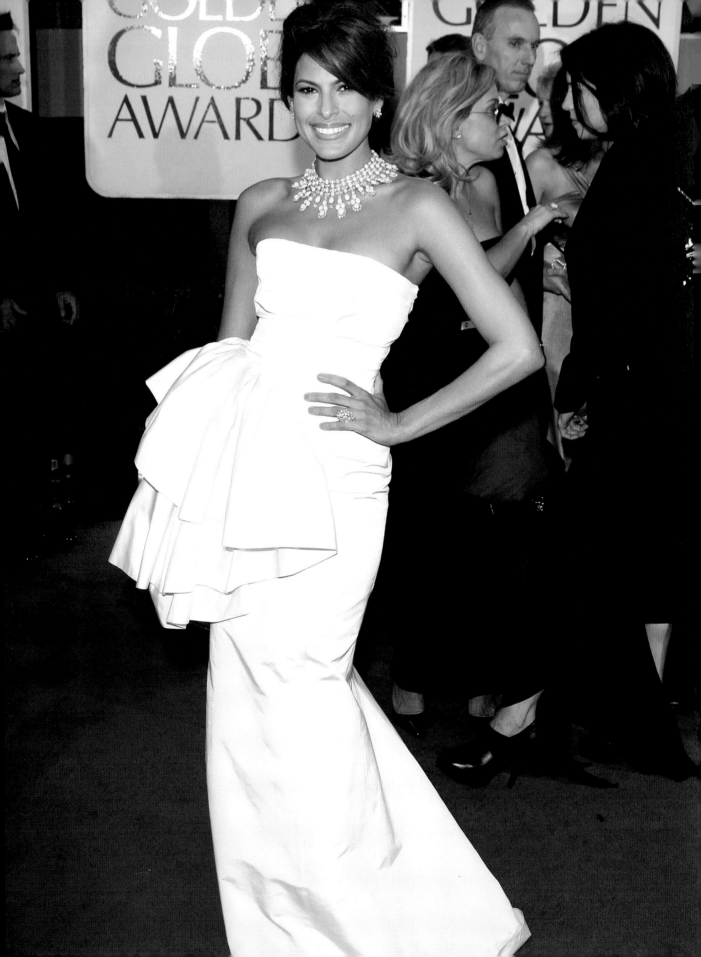

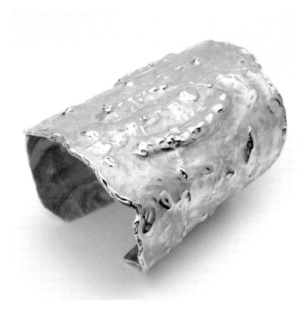

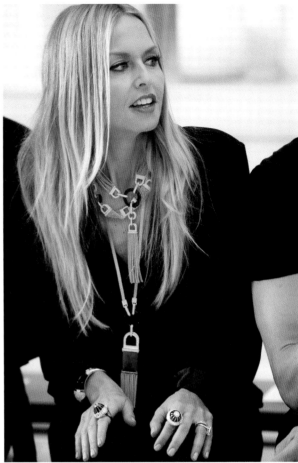

Opposite: Eva Mendes in Dior Haute Couture and a Van Cleef & Arpels necklace, Golden Globes, 2009. This page, clockwise from top left: Van Cleef & Arpels' "Jackie O" cuff; in Rachel Zoe Collection jewelry; Cartier's Panthere ring.

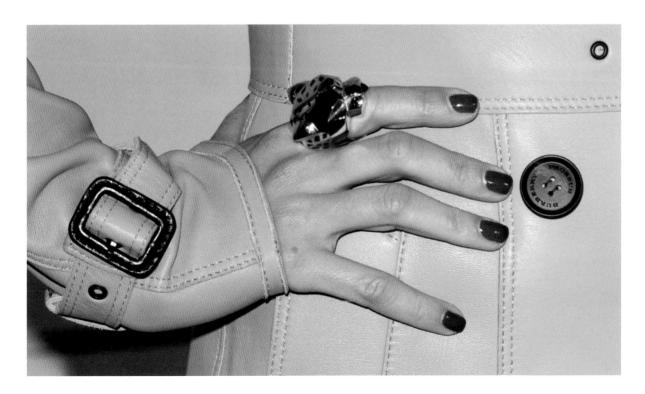

PRECIOUS CARGO

Once you have determined your jewelry persona, the fun really begins; you have a focus when you shop. As a collector of fine and costume jewelry, I am always looking for architectural pieces and those with unique embellishments. Many of my most cherished bracelets and necklaces—like a Lanvin interchangeable jade or tiger-eye pendant and a pair of vintage Dior crystal cuffs—are plated and studded with simple stones.

Before I became a mom, my jewelry philosophy could be summed up as: More is more. I often layered a half-dozen chains around my neck and adorned my wrists and fingers with chunky gold panther rings, snake cuffs, and sometimes even angled pieces with studs. Clearly, you can't hug a toddler if you're wearing a spiked piece of jewelry. Now, I rely on one or maybe two dramatic pieces in my everyday style, like a vintage gold Givenchy circle pendant on a heavy link chain. I think this mandatory lifestyle edit has forced me to become even more creative about my choices.

When it comes to rules, I really have only one "don't": If your ears are pierced, don't forget to wear earrings always—even just a simple pair of studs. Seeing an unadorned hole in an earlobe is just a personal pet peeve of mine; it looks so odd. I'm all for mixing metals like yellow gold with silver or even rose gold and for wearing pieces from different decades. (When it comes to hardware on bags and shoes, however, I like to see unity in gold or silver. More on that later.) I sometimes pair my bold YSL gold chain from the seventies with a pair of classic diamond studs. What I love most about jewelry is that if you're suddenly not feeling a piece, you can just take it off.

LESLIE ROSENZWEIG ON COLLECTING VINTAGE JEWELRY

How do I know Rachel inherited my love for accessories? Since she was ten or eleven, she would take pieces from my collection of jewelry and say, "Oh, Mom will never miss this." Little by little, things would disappear. When she first started styling, she used many of my accessories, such as antique clutches and bracelets on her clients. I once saw Keira Knightley wearing my vintage earrings in a magazine!

I began buying dramatic jewelry in the seventies, when I was in my early twenties. My husband had started an international company and we would often visit Europe—particularly Paris—on business. I always went to a little shop on the Left Bank called Utilité Bébé to pick up runway-inspired costume jewelry that was more affordable than pieces by Dior and Yves Saint Laurent.

As with vintage clothing, Rachel invests only in special designer jewelry that bears a signature or stamp. That label usually means the piece was manufactured in limited edition or sold as high-end costume or fine jewelry—and typically, a piece like that will appreciate in value. But if you're collecting for yourself and don't necessarily look at pieces as investments, you can buy anything and enjoy it. Early on, I collected Miriam Haskell jewelry just because I liked her shapes and ornate styles. I gave a lot of them to Rachel, and now, they are worth a lot more. My taste ran to statement earrings and bracelets that resembled artwork. I loved dramatic pieces and looked for original designs and interesting shapes.

I got to know one vintage dealer named Sandi Berman very well and she supplied me with many wonderful bracelets, necklaces, and earrings. She now owns a fantastic shop in New York on the Upper East Side called Catwalk Couture. I recommend you find a dealer or a shop and buy regularly from that source. The dealer will look for pieces that he or she knows you like and you might even get better deals. Nowadays, the price of vintage jewelry by designers such as Chanel and YSL is outrageous.

I have found interesting pieces at antique shows and flea markets where vendors have booths full of great jewelry. My best advice for finding pieces, signed or not, is to go to country fairs where people are selling estate pieces. I still buy for Rachel every now and again and she still "borrows" whenever she comes home to visit. ■

In 2012, Tiffany & Co. asked me to decorate five different windows at their Fifth Avenue flagship store to celebrate the history of Hollywood glamour from the 1930s through the 1970s. My creations were displayed at Tiffany boutiques around the world. Never mind the fact that this was a dream-come-true opportunity, it also turned out to be an educational experience. To convey the spirit of each era, I explored Tiffany's vast archives and studied the jewelry innovations and design trends within each decade. And I often use what I learned—from how to recognize certain date and purity hallmarks to what innovations came about in design—when I shop for vintage jewelry, fine or costume.

1920s: This is easily one of my favorite decades for jewelry. Deco pieces never become dated. The liberated fashion of the Prohibition era created the need for modern styles of jewelry. Women who bobbed their hair wanted long, sleek geometric earrings and lots of clanking bangles to adorn their newly bare arms. Coco Chanel wore a mismatched pair of black and white earrings in 1926 and started a trend in asymmetrical sets. Because of the discovery of King Tut's tomb in 1922, Egyptian influences were reflected in jewelry's carved gemstones, garland curves, and exotic pharaoh motifs. Cartier's Trinity ring—interlocking yellow, white, and rose gold bands—debuted in 1924 and the style encouraged women to mix metals. Almost a century later, it's still wildly popular and has spurred plenty of similar styles.

Look for: Long necklaces studded with faux pearls or lariats finished with tassels; resin bangles, cuffs, and earrings featuring jade, coral, and onyx. Check out hair ornaments like tiaras and bandeaus worn lower on the forehead.

1930s: The 1929 stock market crash and subsequent Depression put a dent in spending. Costume jewelry was marketed to be worn for just one or two seasons and then tossed away. Can you imagine? Luckily, many of the well-crafted pieces like faux pearl and paste chokers, marcasite pins, and celluloid armlets remain today. The same applies for cuffs that feature huge natural stones. I'm always surprised by their quality and creativity, too.

Look for: I love sparkly clip brooches, which often come in pairs to be worn on the straps of a dress, and elegant compacts inlaid with enamel and gemstones. Swarovski crystals for jewelry date back to the thirties, so seek out lozenge-sized faceted stones in earrings, necklaces, and rings.

1940s: As the popularity of cinema hit an all-time high, Hollywood glamour took hold of the nation, and huge feminine bows, knots, ballerinas, and floral motifs appeared in brooches and bracelets. Van Cleef & Arpels introduced its signature snowflake diamond designs in rings, necklaces, and earrings. Cocktail party trends called for oversized rings with semiprecious stones. Just look at any screen siren of that decade—Ava Gardner, Bette Davis—and you'll see bold diamond earrings and tiered jeweled necklaces.

Look for: Huge topaz and citrine rings that overtake your hand in rose gold mounts and links; ruby and diamond combinations in bands and earrings. Star sapphires and other cabochons or shaped gemstones in rings and pendants are great finds, too.

1950s: Thanks to a savvy marketing campaign for De Beers, diamond engagement rings became de rigueur. And because of their popularity, certificates that graded their quality and value were introduced in 1957. Pearls—both natural and cultured—became all the rage, with fans in Jackie Kennedy and Grace Kelly. Women invested in matching sets of earrings and bracelets and necklaces, rather than in individual pieces. Motifs of the time included animals, bumblebees, butterflies, and flowers—along with the starbursts and Sputniks associated with advances in space exploration. In 1958, America sent its first satellite skyward.

Look for: Highly textural gold pieces with braided and Florentine accents. Abstract modernist midcentury pieces—inspired by Pablo Picasso and Salvador Dalí—in brass or silver make an interesting conversation starter.

1960s: Unconventional elements like uncut crystals and elaborate clawed settings in gold were introduced. Mod pieces in black or white and Day-Glo colors inspired by optical art became the focal point of an outfit in pendants, giant hoop earrings, and multi-strand necklaces.

Look for: Statement button earrings in black or white and huge enamel pendants on snake chains. Thick Lucite cuffs in Day-Glo or saturated colors or with a graphic checkerboard motif.

1970s: The "Me Decade" of individualism brought about a craze for ethnic styles and bold, showy pendants made of horn, bone, and wood. Splashy primary colors seen in enamel pieces mirrored the optimism of Pop Art and disco fever fueled a trend in bright yellow gold. I love the big gold hoops that women wore with their hair straight and parted down the center and lots of bangles on each arm.

Look for: Cool zodiac-inspired pieces and signed costume necklaces by YSL, Givenchy, Lanvin, and Pierre Cardin. Gold or wooden bangles look great in a dramatic stack, and I am always on the lookout for huge link chains and pendants with earthy elements.

Next spread: Windows styled by Rachel Zoe for Tiffany & Co.

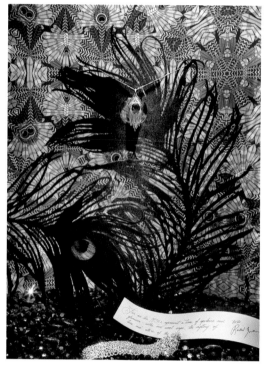

1930s

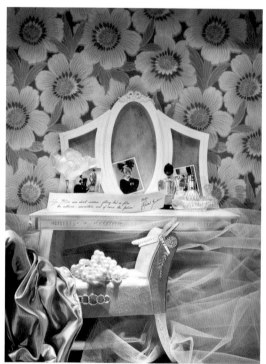

1940s

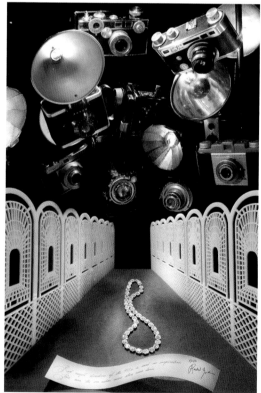

1950s

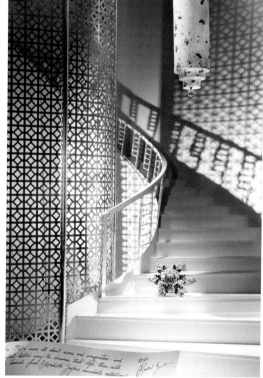

1960s

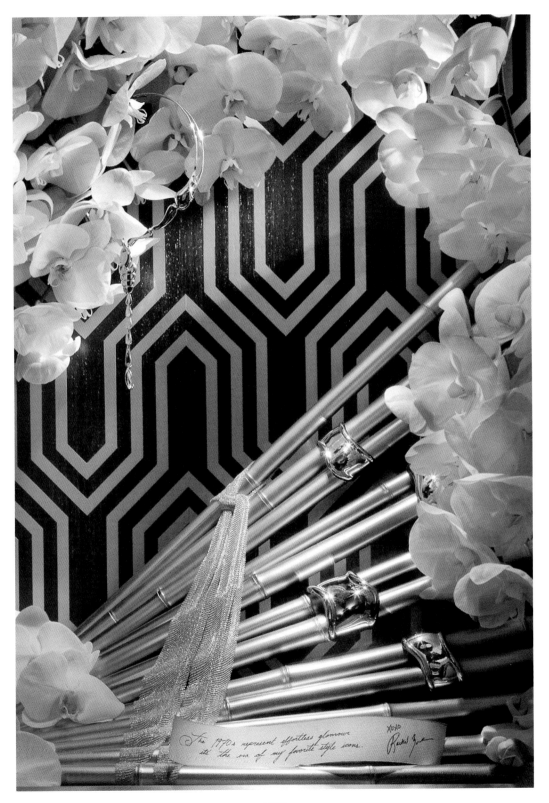

The 1970s represent effortless glamour: it's the era of my favorite style icons.

xoxo
Rachel Zoe

1970s

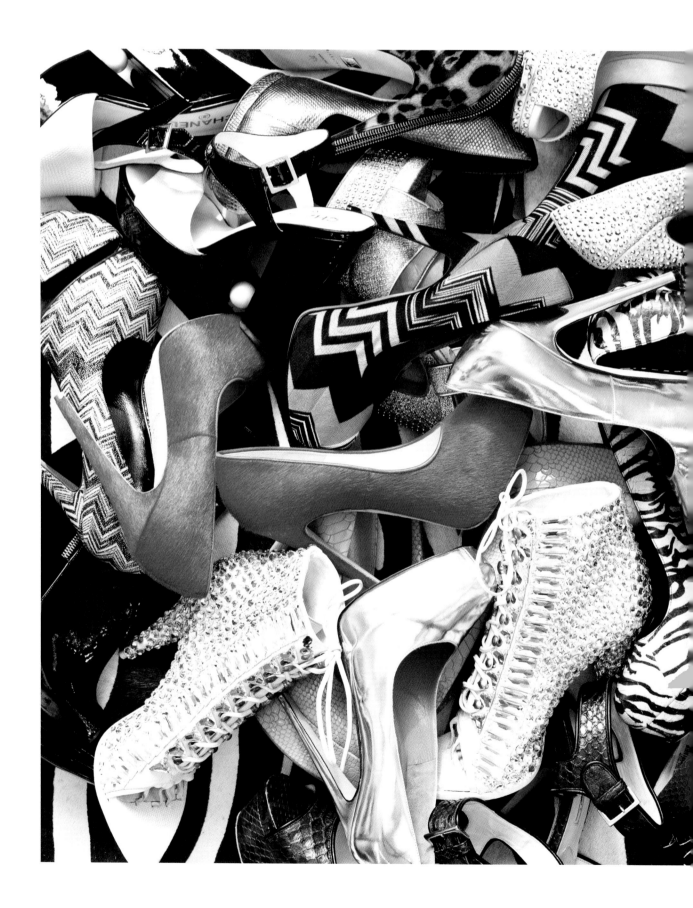

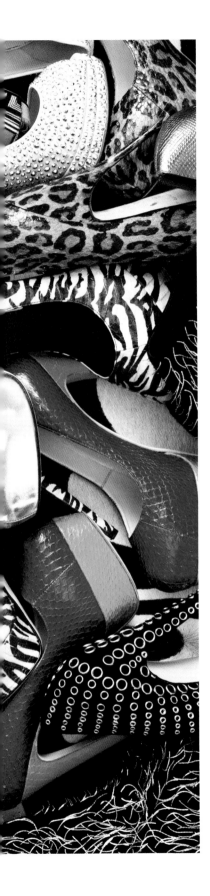

SHOES: THE GREATEST HITS

It's funny that shoes are often the last things we slip on before we head out the door, because women usually notice them first. High heels mean everything to me, because they make me tall. My first were a pair of simple black Charles Jourdan pumps that I snagged from my mom when I was thirteen and I never looked back—and I didn't stumble once either. I swear I was born to wear high heels. My father loves to talk about how athletic I was as a teen. (I played a lot of tennis.) Then, he will laugh and add that I quit sports because I was finally allowed to buy crazy heels and I refused to wear sneakers. He's right!

Now, I don't own a single pair of flats. I even went to the hospital to deliver Skyler in eight-inch Givenchy wedge boots! Yes, I definitely received a few double takes as I teetered into the maternity ward. But it was important for me to feel as chic and pretty as possible as I embarked on the exciting journey to motherhood. It was also the one element of that experience I could control, in a way. And when I left, I was wearing a Halston duster cardigan, floppy hat, big sunglasses, and those same eight-inch heels while cradling my newborn son. By the way, little Sky now has his own share of accents: fedoras, beanies, sunnies, and dozens of pairs of tiny shoes, too. I like to joke that I will accessorize him until the day he puts his foot down and says "No." And on that day, I *at least* know he will be wearing amazing shoes!

Of course, shoes are subjective for everyone—little boys aside. One woman's ballet flat is another's satin stiletto peep-toe. When I design shoes for my collection, I always strive to create classic styles with a little sex appeal—that might be a peek of toe cleavage or a cut that reveals the sensuous line of an arch. In my years of working in fashion, I have developed a sacred list of essential styles that will carry you through any occasion.

BLACK ANKLE BOOT: All hail the bootie. This here-to-stay style of low-cut boot, whether it's a patent platform or a studded suede stiletto, is the new black pump, in my opinion. It can be flat or it can be five inches high. The anklet is modern and versatile, and can infuse a pencil skirt or a little black dress with some edge.

NUDE PUMP: Once again, this shoe will make you love your legs, as they add inches to the line of your silhouette by matching your skin tone. I love to pair nude pumps with minidresses, skinny jeans, and short skirts. Take advantage of their elongating effect and show some skin.

ALL-SEASON WEDGE: What a way to cheat glamour! With a wedge—be it a canvas espadrille or a metallic peep-toe—you get a boost of four to five inches without any discomfort. I rely on them for my busiest days. You can wear this style with a maxi dress, tailored shorts, or even a slim-cut suit. They are amazingly versatile.

RIDING BOOT: There's a reason Gucci has been designing equestrian boots since its inception in 1921. These flat boots that skim just below the knee are both classic and sophisticated. Wear them with skinny jeans and a tweed jacket or a day dress and belted coat. If I weren't petite and determined to be taller than I am, I would wear flat classic riding boots all the time. Thankfully, there are many great high-end and midlevel brands out there with their own versions of the iconic style.

BALLET FLATS: Paired with cropped trousers and a white shirt or a chunky knit, these classic slip-ons always read fresh and youthful. And they remind me of Audrey Hepburn, of course. I love the design of these shoes, because they truly marry fashion and function. Opt for bright colors, embellishments, or even pony hair for a more glamourous finish.

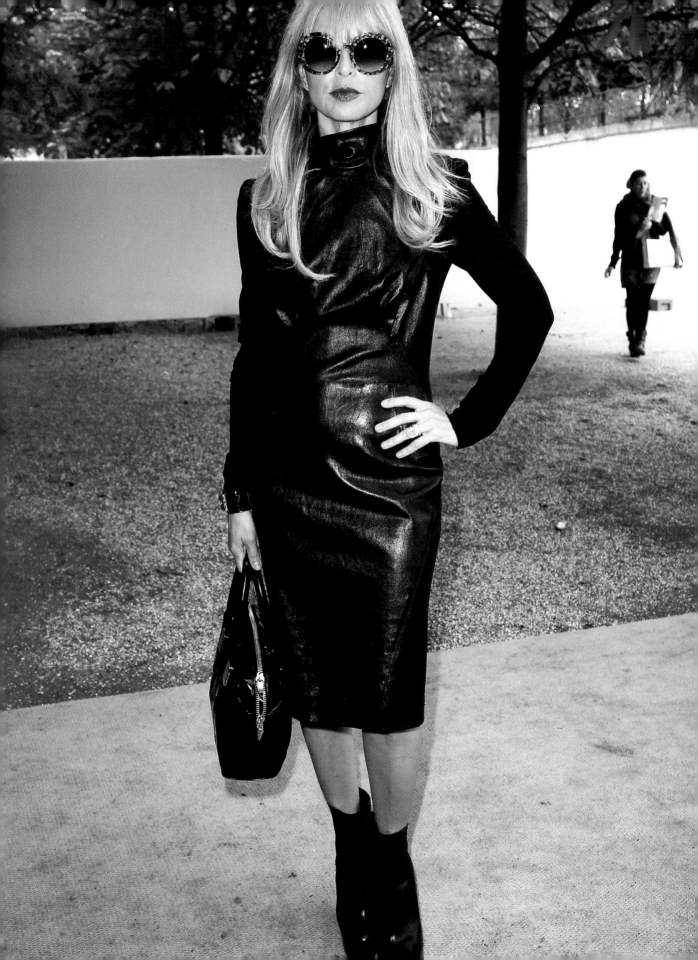

THE ESSENTIAL HANDBAGS

My philosophy on handbags has always been to splurge on a few fantastic investment pieces that you will hopefully own forever—especially since a fabulous handbag can salvage a boring outfit. Besides, cheap leather, hollow hardware, and flimsy construction not only don't last, but are also easy to spot and quickly detract from even the most stylish ensemble. I usually advise against buying the "it" bag of any particular season. A handbag like that can sometimes become passé when a new one takes its place. Of course there are exceptions like the elegantly rounded YSL Muse, Givenchy's Nightingale, Proenza Schouler's chic PS1 satchel, and the uniquely structured Celine Phantom tote. Each of these bags transcends trend in its modern take on an iconic design. But unless you can handle the seasonal splurge, save up for something that's classic and of the best quality you can afford. It doesn't have to be a designer brand either. These are the five styles you should eventually own, because each one will serve you well.

CLUTCH: The options are endless, from a frame to a box to a fold-over to an envelope. Sizes vary, too—small minaudières and oversized clutches that can carry as much as a shoulder bag. I am attracted to a metallic or exotic skin such as python or stingray, because it adds a little drama to any ensemble and works for day or night. You will get the most bang for your buck out of a neutral-hued clutch, but satin or Lucite for special events will get a lot of mileage, as well.

Be sure that: The design you choose can accommodate your necessities. If you're a woman who carries three lipsticks and a spare set of keys, choose accordingly. In fact, it will be helpful to take your essentials with you when you shop for a clutch so you can size correctly.

STRUCTURED TOTE: Depending on your agenda, a sensational tote can land you a business deal or get you through a layover without losing your mind. I opt for black, dark brown, or burgundy—preferably in patent and with feet underneath, as this bag usually takes a beating and often ends up sitting on the floor of a restaurant or plane. Look for one with striking hardware that adds some luxe.

Be sure that: The straps can handle your load. Lugging around a laptop, over time, will wear on the handles and seams—and not to mention your shoulder. Organized pockets, like those for a phone or sunglasses, make it easiest to access everything on the go.

CROSS-BODY OR MESSENGER: Once you go hands free, it can be hard to return to carrying a traditional handbag. If you're a multitasking mom or someone who's constantly on the go, this utilitarian purse will become your chic salvation—especially if it has a smart interior. I always add a cross-body strap to the more classic styles when I'm designing handbags for my collection. Look for soft, luxurious leathers that will wear well over time.

Be sure that: The chain or strap always lies flat. You want the bag itself to sit right above your hipbone and not add unnecessary bulk, so be sure you can adjust it as needed. Most well-designed bags have straps that can be made longer or shorter.

SLOUCHY HOBO: This is the one you'll grab eighty percent of the time—trust me. I thought long and hard before I designed a hobo with a front magnetic snap and an eight-and-a-quarter-inch strap that we tested around the office on women of all different heights. This handbag is really all about the engineering. Gauge the comfort of a few bags, because different shapes and sizes will fall differently on your body.

Be sure that: The body of the bag rests comfortably under your bent elbow. A roomy hobo can easily turn into a black hole, so make certain there are adequate places to stash things you might need to find fast. Or you can use your own individual pouches to keep things organized.

SHOULDER BAG: A ladylike bag always reads grown-up and sophisticated. I like a more structured body with a chain strap, which transforms jeans and a long-sleeved tee into a more polished look. Think of this bag the way you would a tailored jacket and look for great lines and rich embellishments like miniature gold padlocks or horse bits.

Be sure that: This retro-inspired silhouette doesn't look too fussy if you opt to buy vintage. Color blocking, animal prints, and exotic skins will make it feel younger and more modern.

Next page, top: Carrying a Ferragamo clutch. Bottom: A line up of clutches from my closet. Opposite: Carrying a structured Hermès Kelly bag, Fashion Week 2011.

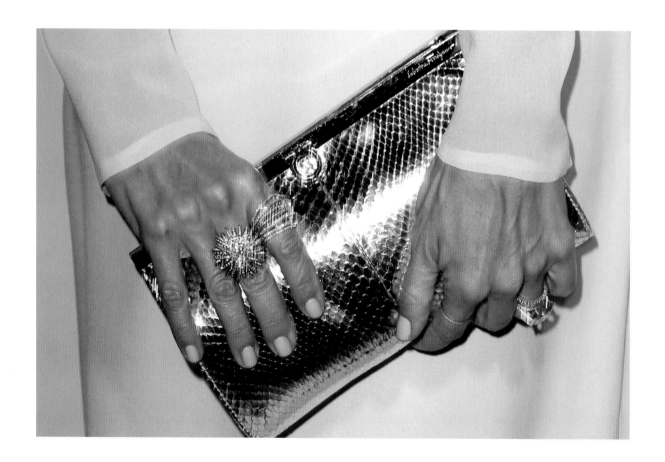

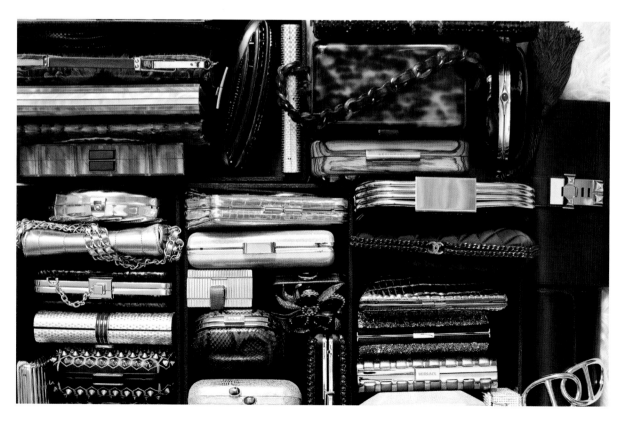

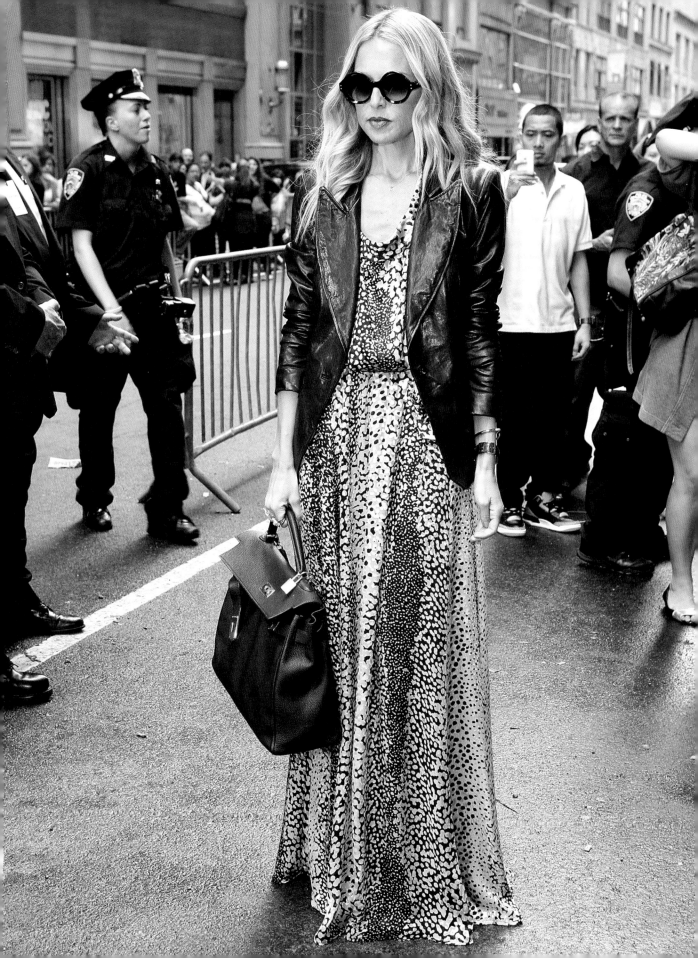

IT'S A CINCH

Never underestimate the power of a belt. Not only will a well-placed one spotlight your waist, but it can also change up the entire look of an outfit. I love the bold contrast of a wide black leather belt with grommets on a classic khaki trench coat, or the texture a skinny strip of snakeskin can lend to a silk sheath. Belts are often the forgotten accessory. I know women who own dozens of pairs of shoes and just one or two belts. You certainly don't need an armload of them; a few key styles will suffice.

WIDE CINCH: Typically about three inches in width, this belt always accentuates your curves and can even add a bold splash of color to an outfit. I love to pair a corsetlike leather one with a pencil skirt or add an elastic knit style with embellishments to a fit and flare dress.

HIP BELT: Worn low, this belt instantly delivers polish to a pair of low-rise jeans or a tunic and lengthens the torso. A thick brown braided one with a bold brass buckle reads classic with white jeans and a sailor stripe sweater. I love to anchor a maxi dress with a hip belt that has some serious hardware.

SKINNY BELT: Trust me when I say that this delicate belt can be your style savior. Whether it's a thin classic alligator style, one with brushed grommets, or even a simple patent leather, a skinny belt can dress up or add dimension to everything from high-waist jeans to a pencil skirt to a long knit cardigan. An animal print version or bright, colorful lizard belt makes a little black dress pop, too.

CHAIN BELT: In 1956, Chanel popularized this rich look of what is, in essence, a statement necklace worn around the waist—preferably with a few dangling charms or even a dozen faux gold coins. Vintage Chanel and YSL chain-link belts are always super glamourous, but you can also find non-designer gold chain belts threaded with leather that work just as well, or any long, bold link necklace can easily double as one, too. A fitted, ribbed black turtleneck with white pants and a gold chain belt is classic perfection.

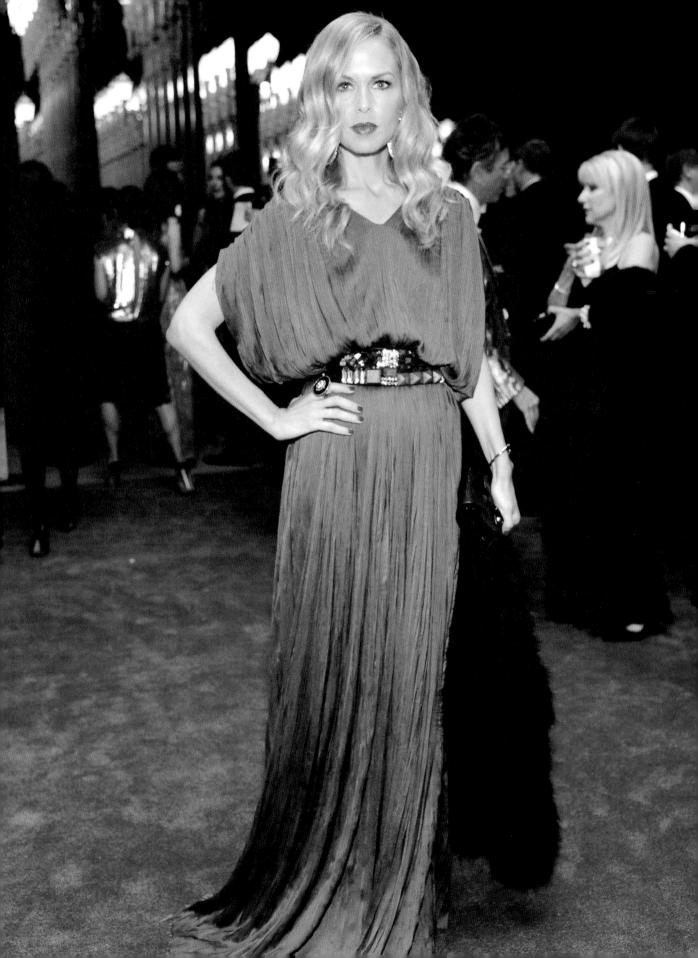

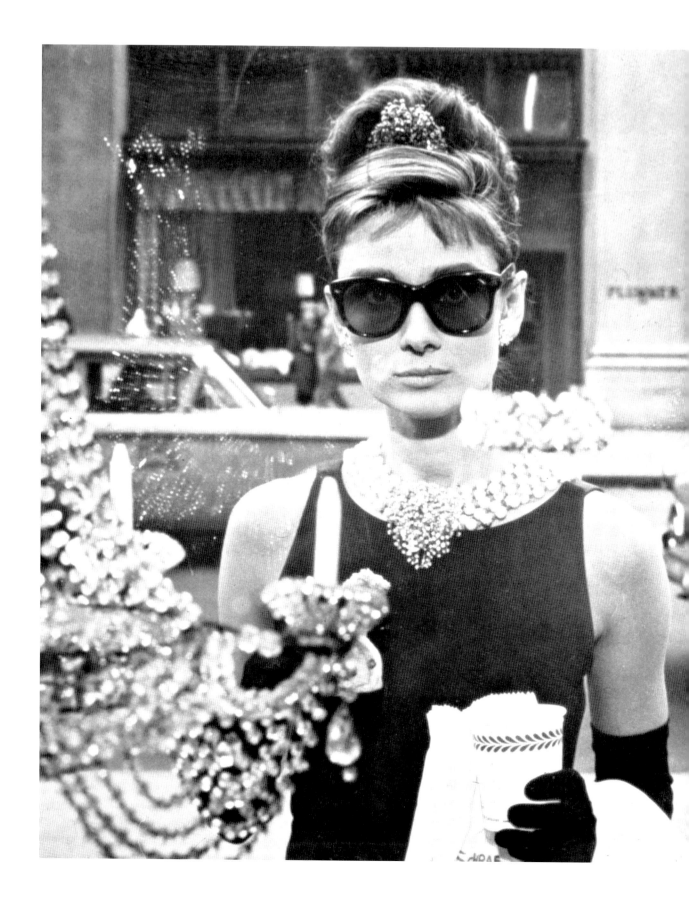

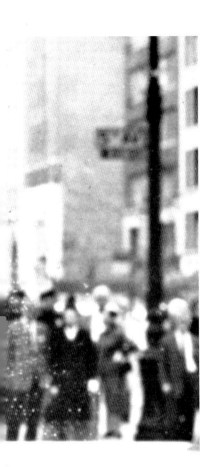

OPTICAL OBSESSION

In my opinion, sunglasses can make just as much of a statement as jewelry—I never leave home without two pairs. They can disguise the aftermath of a late night, or just allow you to be a little mysterious. I like to think of sunnies as "do not disturb" signs. Plus, a fabulous pair of shades can upgrade a simple look to super stylish and sophisticated.

My addiction to sunglasses might explain why I have three drawers filled with them in my closet! Here in Los Angeles, shades are essential—especially since my light green eyes are extremely sensitive to bright light. When I'm in a rush to get out the door, I rely on big dark sunglasses and bold red lipstick for instant glamour. And unless I'm wearing a semitransparent lens, I always remove them inside. When it comes to choosing a frame, it's important you set aside time to try on at least a dozen pairs. My favorite frames have distinctly different personalities and I rotate them depending on my mood or outfit. Some busy days call for an easy, casual look with aviators, while a pair of oversized dark frames can make a sleek suit look even more cosmopolitan.

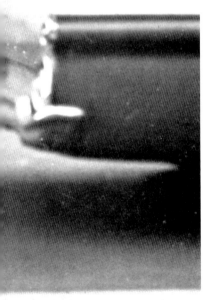

WAYFARER: Being a fan of midcentury architecture, I love that this style was designed to reflect the cool minimalism of Charles Eames. And the fact that Bob Dylan, John F. Kennedy, and Audrey Hepburn all wore them says it all. Bold colored frames are fun for a contemporary take on this classic look.

Audrey Hepburn

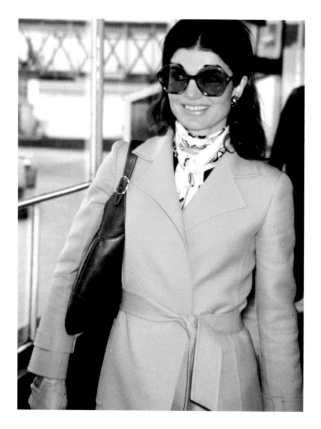

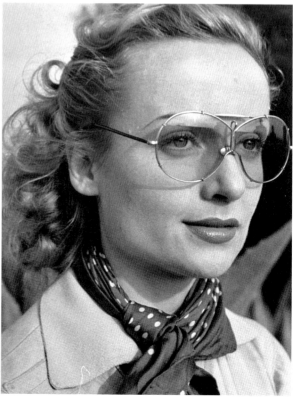

OVERSIZED: There is just no faster or easier way to access high-impact glamour than slipping on a pair of huge sunnies—and this is the style that you'll catch me in most often. Jackie Onassis actually commissioned Nina Ricci and Parisian optical designer François Pinton to create unique oversized frames for her back in the 1960s. Clearly, she knew they would help camouflage her identity, but I suspect she knew she would start a trend, too.

AVIATOR: These lightweight teardrop-shaped specs convey classic cool and exude a sense of adventure—they were originally developed by Ray-Ban for pilots in 1936. You can experiment with the lens size, hue, and material of frame. I love the traditional gold metal with a dark green lens, but you should also check out tortoiseshell or horn frames with blue, yellow, or even a mirrored lens. I'm forever a fan of Ray-Bans, too.

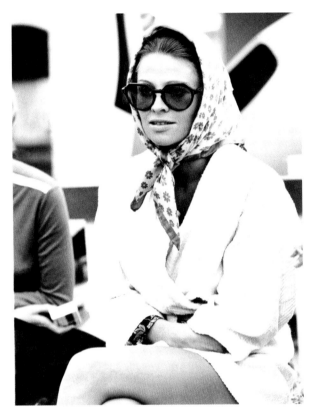

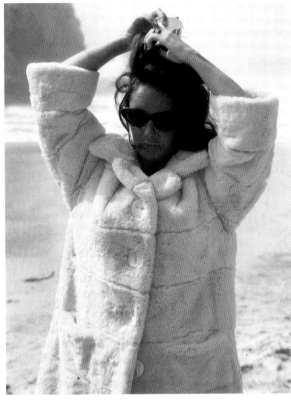

ROUND: What can I say about a style that both Coco Chanel and John Lennon popularized in their day? They can read either mod hippie or gamine chic, depending on your outfit. Wear them in the compact size of a silver dollar or go as huge and dramatic as Elton John, which I have done on many occasions. I love an ombré lens with an acetate or Lucite frame.

CAT-EYE: For me, this shape summons the glamour of the fifties with visions of Marilyn Monroe and Elizabeth Taylor. If the pointed eyes feel too retro, choose a subtler take on the shape with a rounder version. Or go all out and over-the-top with an animal print frame.

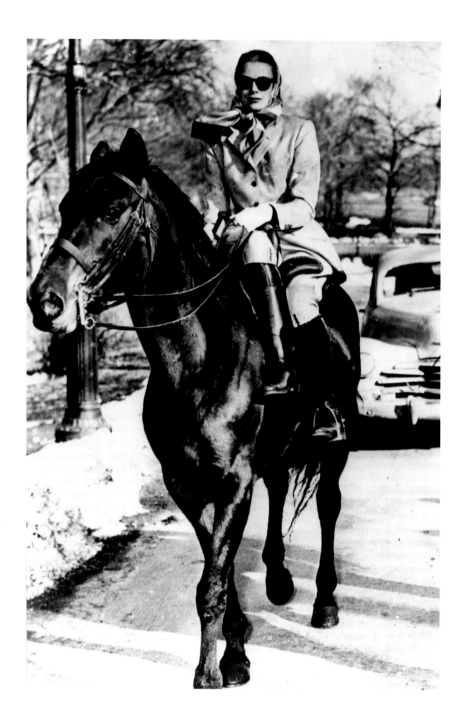

TIE ME UP

Hermès sells one of its signature scarves every twenty-five seconds, which is no surprise to me. The iconic silk square, with its plump hand-rolled hems, has become one of the most versatile accessories since it debuted in 1937—so versatile that Grace Kelly wore one as a chic sling when she broke her arm in 1956, while Sharon Stone multitasked with the scarf in a bondage scene in *Basic Instinct.* But one of my favorite interpretations of the scarf comes courtesy of Madonna, who wore one as a bandeau top in *Swept Away.*

But you don't have to splurge on designer scarves. I'm always on the lookout for fantastic prints—whether it's the Pucci-inspired geometrics of the fifties or a vivid colorful floral—when I visit vintage shops or flea markets. And there are plenty of styles beyond the classic silk scarf. Long skinny knit scarves, chunky wool ones, fur stoles, and larger cashmere wraps can refine any look, too. I love a fringe, an animal print, or bold colored knit to add a point of interest. There are so many ways to wear one.

BEACH DAY: A vibrant scarf looks fantastic and ultra-glamourous at the beach, especially when you wear it with a black, white, or neutral bathing suit. Fold the scarf into a triangle and wear it pirate- or handkerchief-style with soft beach waves or a long braid.

JOB INTERVIEW: The classic button-down white shirt and fitted blazer get upgraded to elegant with a colorful scarf worn tucked inside the shirt-front like an ascot. It's a great way to show some personality and style to a potential employer, while still being conservative enough to come off as professional.

FIRST DATE: When the scarf is folded into a tie and worn as a sixties-style headband, it always reads mod and feminine with a touch of innocence. Look for a pop of color that contrasts with your hair.

BUSINESS DINNER: Europeans have mastered the pull through, and it's an effortlessly chic way to wear any scarf. Simply fold a scarf in half and tug the ends through the U of the loop. You're set! Wear it with a fitted knit cardigan and pencil skirt or more casually, underneath a peacoat.

WINTER STROLL: Thicker scarves, fur stoles or collars, and large cashmere wraps not only prevent a chill but also add a vibrant, textural layer to a black, camel, or winter-white coat. I like to wear an oversized, featherweight cashmere scarf since the volume of the fabric adds interest to any winter coat. Wraps can look a bit dated if worn like shawls, so I artfully drape one so that one end sits just over the shoulder.

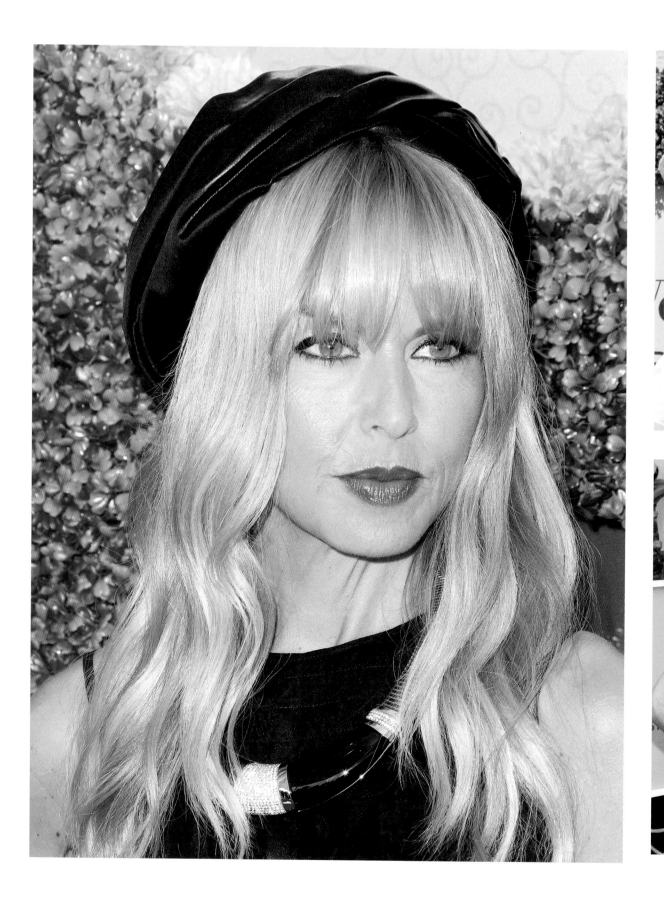

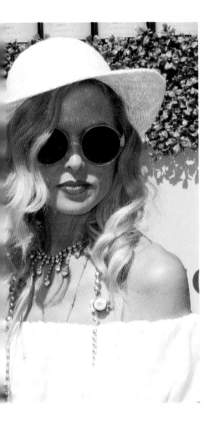

TOP IT OFF

Hats are such an easy shortcut to chic. I think part of their appeal for me is the fact that so few people wear them nowadays. I'm not talking about baseball caps, of course—my taste veers toward sophisticated felted fedoras that inject a dash of androgyny, or a faux fur fez that makes you look totally jet set. Just donning a hat makes a statement in itself. When a woman walks into a restaurant in a great ivory linen suit with a jaunty Panama, everyone stops and looks her way. It feels almost cinematic.

My own personal hat collection runs the gamut from black oversized floppy ones banded with grosgrain ribbon to chunky knit gray cashmere beanies. I love the elegance and simplicity of a cloche, which adds an elegant deco touch to modern skinny jeans and a cropped jacket. Some women say that they don't look good in hats, or that they don't feel comfortable in them. My philosophy on wearing hats is, the more you sport them, the more you grow to love them. Experiment with different brims and shapes; there is a style out there for everyone. To add a little flair to a hat band (the edging just above the inner-brim), I sometimes pin on a vintage pearl brooch or a couple of pheasant feathers. You can even circle a skinny belt around the band to add some texture or a pop of color, too.

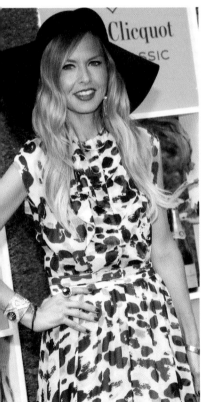

Clockwise from left: In a vintage Dior turban. In a vintage straw fedora. In a Rachel Zoe Collection hat.

As a designer, I incorporate my hats into every runway show. For a Spring presentation, a model might wear a raffia newsboy cap with a sleek denim shorts suit. It's a hat style that can read casual with denim and a cardigan or dressed up with a floral day dress. A black floppy straw hat on a model in an ethereal white dress for spring screams "South of France!" I wear mine whenever I hit the beach. For autumn, I love a structured felt fedora, like the one I paired with a gray plaid, slim-cut suit for my Fall 2012 collection. The hat lends a little tomboy street cool to a ladylike silhouette. But probably one of my favorite looks is the Russian fur hat. As you probably guessed, my inspiration for it was Julie Christie in *Doctor Zhivago*. If you live in a climate that calls for one of these amazing—and warm—hats, go for it.

GET A GRIP

Don't forget your fingers! Gloves, too, can make an equally stylish statement. I own a small stockade of leather gloves in rich earth tones such as caramel and mahogany. I love anything in suede, leather, embossed, or crocodile. The shot of texture and color looks elegant peeking out from the three-quarter sleeves of a winter-white cocoon coat or the cuffs of a traditional cashmere cardigan. Studded black leather gloves or even fingerless ones imbue a ladylike look with a little grit and edge.

Honestly, mittens are not part of my cold weather accessories repertoire. They are too bulky for me—and how does one text? Muffs, on the other hand, couldn't be more elegant and retro chic, whether in faux or real fur. A muff is one of those accessories you may question initially, but wear one on a chilly day and you'll be collecting compliments.

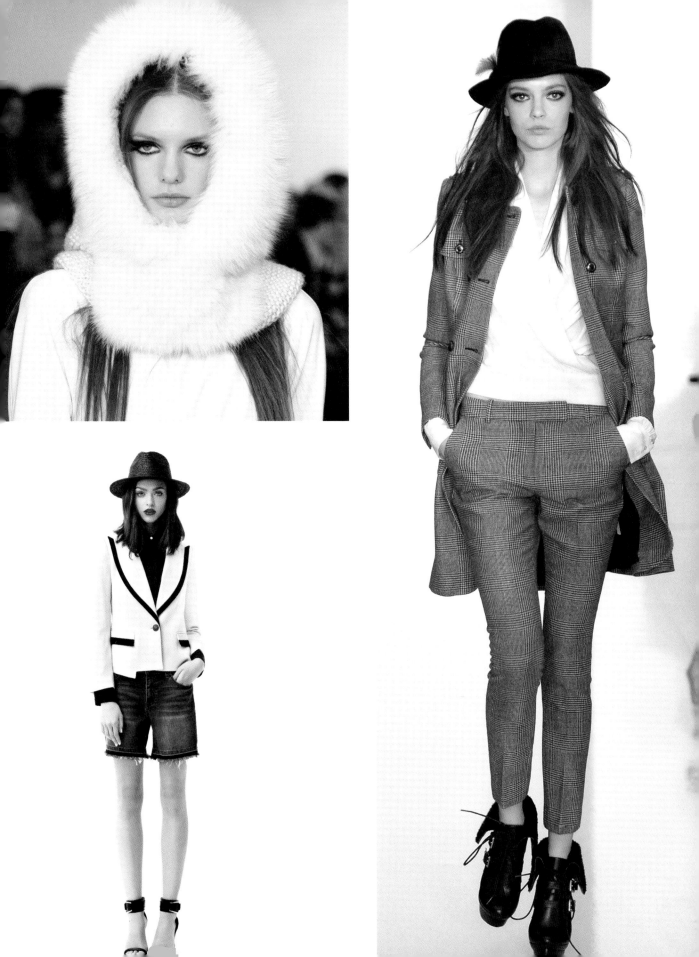

GETTING GORGEOUS

People may compliment your shoes or bag, but their gaze will invariably settle on your face. And while a dramatic red pout will make you stand out in a crowd, it's all that you radiate in that split-second of being noticed that counts. My philosophy on beauty is that it comes more from an inner confidence than from any cosmetic. If you feel fantastic, you look it. You don't need to smile at your reflection whenever you pass a mirror — but you definitely shouldn't scowl either. Admire yourself. Appreciate yourself.

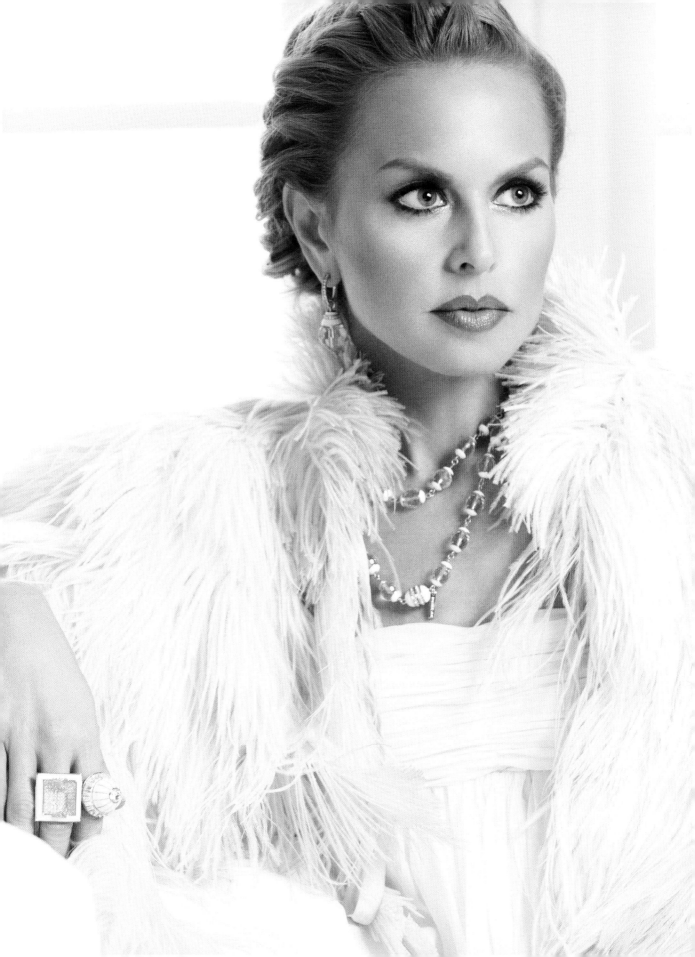

THE ALLURE OF ASYMMETRY

Perfection has never appealed to me—especially when it comes to beauty. What you may perceive as an imperfection can actually become an asset. I love to see a gap in the front teeth, à la Lauren Hutton. Fun fact: Hutton refused to succumb to pressure from modeling agencies to fill the space in her smile and went on to land the very first million-dollar contract with Revlon in 1974. And Cindy Crawford's beauty mark—which was airbrushed off her debut cover for *British Vogue*—has become as much a part of her natural beauty as her insanely high cheekbones and beautiful smile.

> "MY PHILOSOPHY ON BEAUTY IS THAT IT COMES MORE FROM AN INNER CONFIDENCE THAN FROM ANY COSMETIC. IF YOU FEEL FANTASTIC, YOU LOOK IT."

When I admire someone's looks, it's always because of a standout feature. Maybe it's a strong jawline that accentuates a full mouth, or wide-set eyes that make the composition of a face all the more arresting. A sincere smile can make a pronounced difference, too. Even in choosing models for my own runway shows, I am not seeking complete symmetry or an utterly perfect profile. What's more fascinating to me is a confident gaze and sense of self that comes with appreciating your own beauty.

If you look in the mirror and find yourself focusing on a high forehead or a crooked nose, you're overlooking the entire package. I always say with a laugh that I have oversized features—big lips, big cheeks, big eyes. But I embrace what I have and focus on enhancing my assets. Take a peek at your own face and do the same. Instead of zeroing in on your least favorite features and trying to downplay them, focus on what you love and play up those areas.

Love your lips? Make them the focal point of your face with a statement red, coral, or berry. If you want to highlight your eyes, begin your makeup routine by emphasizing them with mascara and bold liner so that

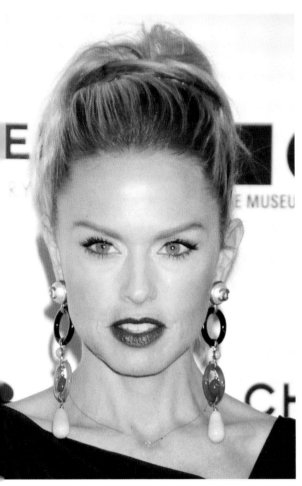

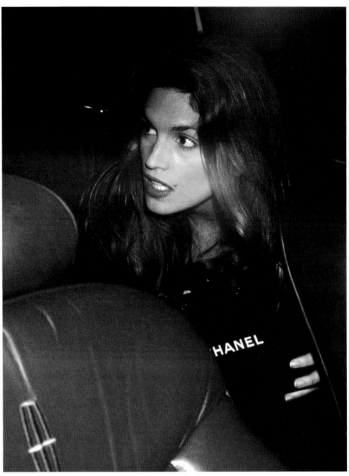

"PERFECTION HAS NEVER APPEALED TO ME—
ESPECIALLY WHEN IT COMES TO BEAUTY.
WHAT YOU MAY PERCEIVE AS AN IMPERFECTION
CAN ACTUALLY BECOME AN ASSET."

they take center stage. Amazing cheekbones deserve a dab of shimmer to accentuate their contours. The same applies to hair. You can spotlight shine with a pin-straight style or underscore your mane's untamable nature with sexy beach waves. Once you start focusing on your best feature, it will quickly become the first thing you notice when you spot your reflection in the mirror.

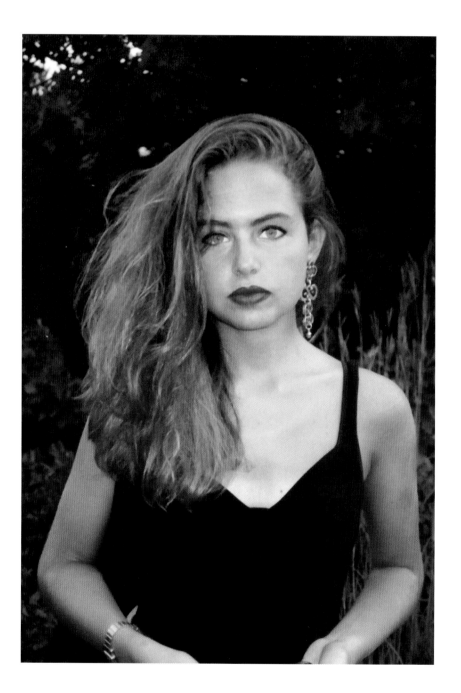

ABOUT FACE

You might think you need to use more makeup as you get older, but the opposite is true. I wear about half as much now as I did when I was a teenager. Back in the horrifying eighties, I went overboard with the Sun In and frosty pink lipstick. When I look at photographs from that era, I shudder. How did I not see that a head of brassy highlights and turquoise eyeliner aged me a decade?

In those days, taking care of my skin was hardly a priority. I rarely washed off my makeup before I went to bed, let alone applied any sort of moisturizer. At this point in my life, you would never catch me wearing a smoky eye from the night before in the morning. I'm obsessive about cleansing, exfoliating, and adding moisturizer to every inch of my face and body. If you spent a day with me, you would see me applying hand lotions and lip balm almost every hour. You should think of your skin as your most important investment; you can grab a chic fedora to disguise a bad hair day, but no amount of concealer or foundation will camouflage neglected skin.

"YOU MIGHT THINK YOU NEED TO USE MORE MAKEUP AS YOU GET OLDER, BUT THE OPPOSITE IS TRUE. I WEAR ABOUT HALF AS MUCH NOW AS I DID WHEN I WAS A TEENAGER."

In Chapter 2, I talked about my uniform—that go-to outfit that never lets me down. I have one for beauty as well. My reliable everyday look always centers on a fresh, healthy complexion and I alternate between a statement lip and a dramatic eye. Through experience, I have learned these will fight for attention on your face. That's never good. I pick one, like a matte berry pout or cat-eye, and then make that emphasis the point of interest on my face. How to decide which? It all depends on the day. If I know that my schedule calls for running around the city and I want to look more glamourous than I feel, I apply a bright red lip and add huge sunnies. Meanwhile, a statement eye with bold liner and mascara serves me better at important meetings where I'm making eye contact with a lot of people.

"YOU SHOULD THINK OF YOUR SKIN AS YOUR MOST IMPORTANT INVESTMENT; YOU CAN GRAB A CHIC FEDORA TO DISGUISE A BAD HAIR DAY, BUT NO AMOUNT OF CONCEALER OR FOUNDATION WILL CAMOUFLAGE NEGLECTED SKIN."

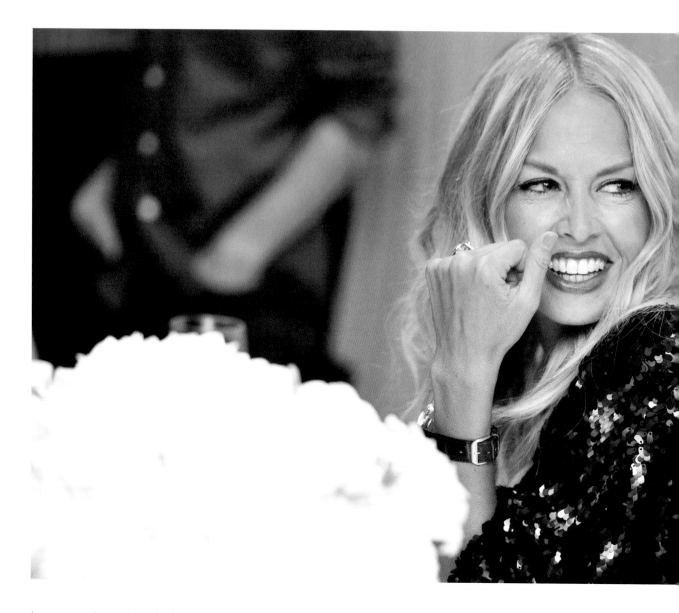

In my everyday makeup look

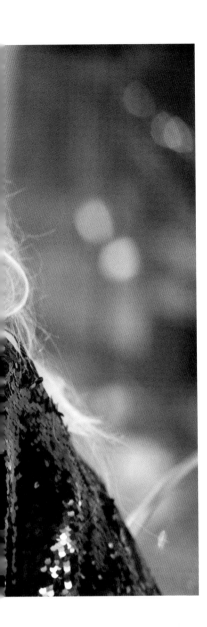

I always keep a few day-to-night necessities at my office — and in my car — for a quick transformation. I add another coat of mascara and thicken my eyeliner or slightly smudge it for a smoky effect; I dab a little shimmer on my cheekbones, and finally, I deepen my lip, whether it's taking it from a pinky brown to a plum or overlaying vibrant red with a vampy Bordeaux shade.

"MY RELIABLE EVERYDAY LOOK ALWAYS CENTERS ON A FRESH, HEALTHY COMPLEXION AND I ALTERNATE BETWEEN A STATEMENT LIP AND A DRAMATIC EYE."

My day and night looks definitely vary depending upon my mood, but I never veer too far from my goal of looking effortlessly glamourous. Some women have made their distinctive beauty choices a personal trademark. Think of Gwen Stefani with her vivid red lips and platinum blond pompadour. I love this story: Gwen's grandmother gave her a crimson lipstick in high school and she has been fiercely loyal to the color ever since. Or Jennifer Lopez, who always radiates a natural sensuality with her light chestnut tresses, flawless complexion, and nude lips.

Finding your signature look is just a matter of practice and patience. I should know. After years of flirting with caramel highlights, I finally went honey blond a few years ago. And every once in a while, I try on a lipstick shade that's the complete opposite of my usual hue — that's how I discovered my love for a deep plum. Experimenting is exciting. Be bold. Have fun. Define beauty in your own way.

JOEY MAALOUF'S THREE EASY STEPS TO FLAWLESS SKIN

I share Rachel's fixation with radiant skin. Luckily, you can cheat a bit and get there with the right products and tricks. While you might think you should test your foundation on your wrist or jawline, your décolletage is really the best match for skin. This way, your face and body colors won't clash or be off at all. When choosing a color for your base products, always be sure to match the shade in natural light.

> "EXPERIMENTING IS EXCITING. BE BOLD. HAVE FUN. DEFINE BEAUTY IN YOUR OWN WAY."

For a flush of color that stays put until you wash your face—and you had better wash that face before bed!—opt for cream blush. Unlike powder, it blends right into the foundation and actually stains the skin. Don't be afraid of vibrant cream pinks and peaches. These go on sheerer than they appear and tone down with blending, complementing your skin's glow.

To finalize your look after you've filled in the details, colorless finishing powder, loose or pressed, goes on invisibly and will set your foundation all day. The minerals also absorb any oil or shine and give skin a silky finish. I recommend looking for one in a light reflecting formula for an extra dewy effect. ■

RED-CARPET GLAM

A lipstick shade is as important as a shoe. A coif—whether it's a side-parted high ponytail or a sexy waterfall of waves—should complement a gown as much as a clutch. When I style a client during award season, the fittings don't end with her outfits and accessories. My team—aka "the glam squad"—and I put together a head-to-toe look, because an ensemble requires the right makeup and hair to be really fabulous. I have seen the most stunning dress overshadowed by a messy mane or an overdone smoky eye that clashed with the final aesthetic too many times.

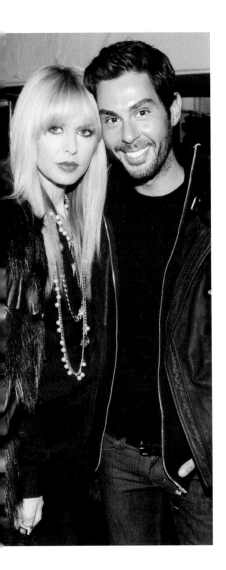

Most of the time, my input on makeup for my clients is instinctual. I'm always partial to a berry lip with dewy skin and major lashes for a formal evening event, or a dramatic topknot that can be softened with loose tendrils. Finding the right hair and makeup isn't a science, but certain elements of a dress should be considered.

COLOR: Matching your eye shadow exactly to your dress is risky business and often reads as too monochromatic. Instead, pick a shade within that color family—for instance, a muted khaki looks fabulous with emerald green. An accent of gold or bronze on your cheeks will break up the color conformity. Any neutral hue on your eye—gray, black, navy, or brown—always complements any jewel-tone or pastel dress. Don't forget the dozens of gorgeous tonal browns to choose from, like fawn, mocha, and nutmeg. Dresses in black or white make the perfect palette for "wow" eye shadow colors like deep purple or even an electric blue liner. Similarly, don't coordinate your lip color exactly to the hue of your dress—go a few shades deeper or lighter.

FABRIC: The weight and texture of your outfit should also dictate your beauty moment. A light silk chiffon or lace look calls for a romantic transparent wash of color rather than major statement makeup. Velvet, leather, brocade, or wool crepe can carry a more dramatic eye or strong lip. You can mimic texture like braiding on a gown in your hair, too. Of course, shine should also be considered. A silk-satin gown looks great with a polished, glossy hairstyle.

DECADE: If you're wearing vintage or a dress inspired by another era, keep your makeup and hair contemporary—at least avoid the over-the-top looks that defined that same time period. Pairing a midcentury mod shift with a dramatic cat-eye and backcombed bouffant will look more costumey than chic. Instead, keep it modern: pin straight and parted down the middle coif or a casual ponytail.

STYLE AND MOVEMENT: Off-duty mini or workplace shirtdress? A minimalist sheath or a flowing macramé maxi dress? Clean lines cry out for similar hair and makeup, like a fresh face and coral or deep plum lip, depending on the season. Also, you don't want to pair a seriously smoky eye with a day dress for the office or an afternoon event. I think a neat side braid or a high, tight ponytail always works with an architectural dress. A long maxi or more ethereal style that floats looks amazing with "Juliet" hair, romantic waves, or a tousled topknot.

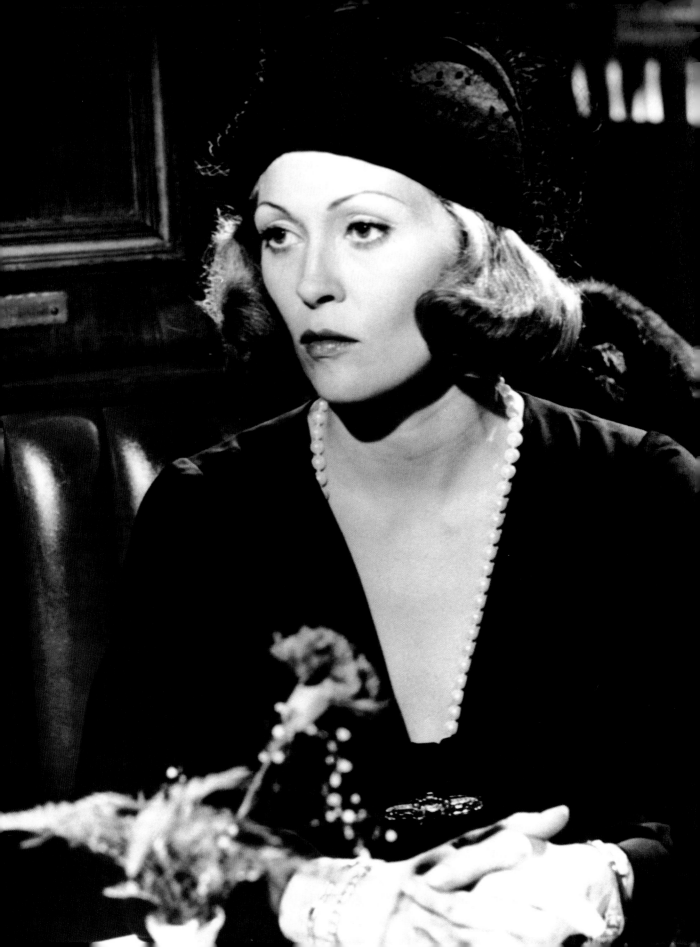

My obsession with vintage doesn't stop at twenties art deco jewelry and mod shifts from the Kennedy era. Beauty trends from previous decades are a great source of inspiration, too. When I contemplate a look, I sometimes scan photos of movie stars like Elizabeth Taylor back in the fifties or Faye Dunaway from *Chinatown* in 1974.

Every decade has its beauty trends and some become more memorable than others. Here's my cheat sheet to the glamour moments worth revisiting from the past.

1920s: The dark berry heart-shaped lip—popularized by the silent screen actress Clara Bow—which overaccentuates the V or cupid's bow of the upper lip. A toned-down version of this bold lip can look totally modern.

1930s: Sultry Greta Garbo popularized the pencil-thin arched brow, which was often drawn on. Lashes were always curled outward and upward, too, which really adds pop—this is my preferred way to accentuate my eyes.

1940s: Pinup glamour took hold in Veronica Lake peekaboo waves and dramatic red lips with matching nails. I can't even tell you how often we re-create old Hollywood for the red carpet, mimicking that look to a tee. You don't need to update this classic.

1950s: Makeup became softer, as Christian Dior introduced pink and coral lipsticks. Liner always had a slight kick to elongate the eye and add subtle drama—a still-fantastic day look now.

1960s: This is one of my favorite eras for beauty, with its emphasis on over-the-top lashes, bold liner, and a pale, nude lip. Monochromatic mod that continues to work now!

1970s: Natural, fresh-faced beauties like Farrah Fawcett brought the focus to bronzed skin, feathered hair, and light makeup. Who didn't want to look like one of Charlie's Angels back in the day? The natural, sun-kissed look is now timeless, thanks to them.

1980s: Big hair and yellow eye shadow aside, the eighties had some redeeming beauty moments, too. Contouring cheeks with blush, bold brows, and navy eyeliner were trends with staying power that I still love.

1990s: Minimalistic beauty—a revolt against eighties excess—ruled the runways and overtook the streets. Sleek chignons and low ponytails replaced big hair; a dewy complexion with a natural flush and scant eye makeup became perfect in its simplicity. This emphasis on the face, which has always encouraged me to take great care of my skin, never goes out of style. It's an unexpected and fresh look for evening, too.

Opposite: Faye Dunaway.

Next spread, top row: Clara Bow, Greta Garbo, Veronica Lake, Sophia Loren. Bottom row: Jean Shrimpton, Farrah Fawcett, Christie Brinkley, Kate Moss.

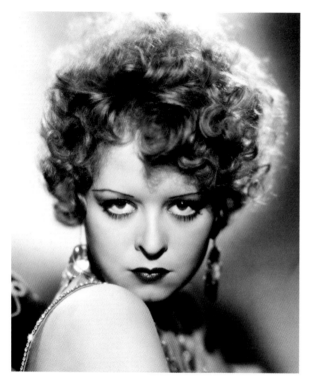

1920s

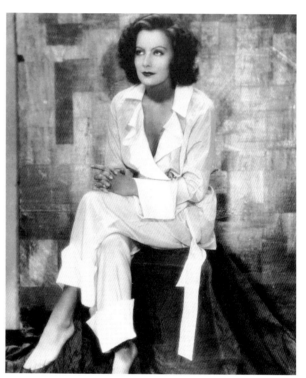

1930s

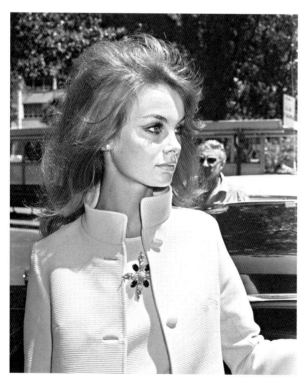

1960s

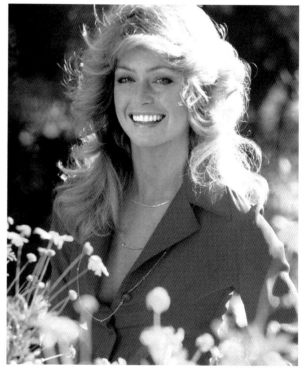

1970s

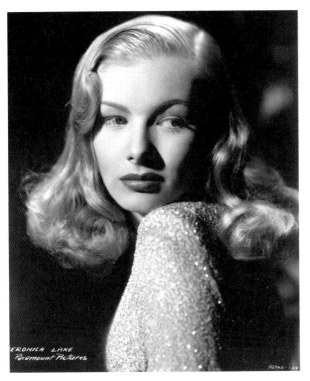

1940s

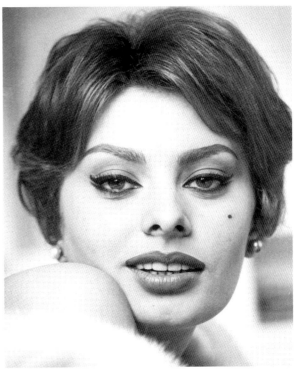

1950s

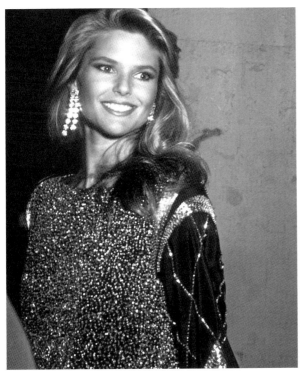

1980s

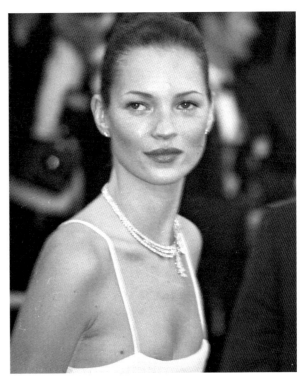

1990s

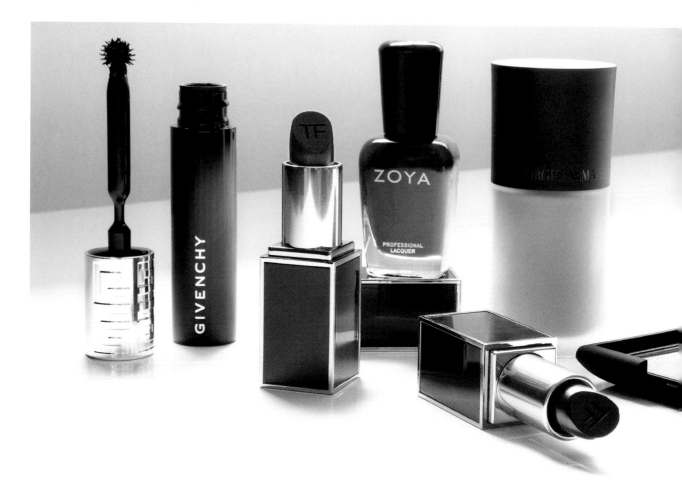

My "hero kit"

YOUR "HERO KIT"

You know the lipstick that always does the trick when you dig it out of your purse for a touch-up? I do. There are products I literally can't live without and I call that collection my "hero kit." My loyalty to these exceptional items is so deep that I buy them in bulk and divvy them up for at-home use, on-the-go touch-ups, and travel. I probably own a half-dozen NARS Orgasm blushes—and I'm okay with that.

Of course, editing can be as crucial as accumulating. Sometimes, you discover your heroes by singling them out of your own collection. Empty out your makeup bag and decide if every product deserves its place. Does your concealer glide on effortlessly and stay put? Do you always achieve the perfect winged eye with that liquid liner? I like to keep the extra products that I use only occasionally in a drawer by my bathroom sink. Every three months or so, I go through the goods and throw away anything that I haven't touched in a while. Unfortunately, makeup usually

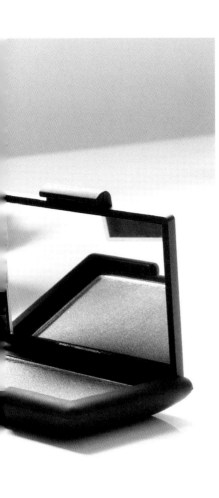

doesn't come with an expiration date, but many products are susceptible to bacteria and lose their effectiveness over time. I'm pretty meticulous about regularly replacing items like mascara, which needs to be changed out at least every three months. Eye and lip pencils can be used for a year as long as you sharpen them every week to keep the tip hygienic. Liquid foundations last about six months before the formula breaks down, while lipsticks and glosses have a lifespan of about a year. I use only organic skincare and body creams, which tend to expire within six months because they don't contain preservatives.

Storage is important, too. There's nothing worse than not being able to zipper a bag shut because of product overload. I stash my "heroes" in a roomy canvas cosmetics pouch that's lined with a material that can be easily cleaned. Here's what you will find inside:

EGYPTIAN MAGIC: Ever since hearing about this moisturizing balm a decade ago, I have been addicted. I use it on my face, my hair, and even dab a little on my leather bags to soften them or remove a stain. It was my go-to product throughout my pregnancy for dry skin.

TATCHA BEAUTY PAPERS: These fragrance- and powder-free blotting sheets are life changing. They remove the oil from your face without smudging your makeup. At the end of the day, I always blot my face before adding more products for an evening event.

NARS ORGASM BLUSH: This peach-pink shade with gold flecks delivers the perfect dose of sun-kissed shimmer on my cheekbones. I even keep a compact in my kitchen for a quick pick-me-up! During the summer, I also use the Multiple version of the product—a cream blusher in a chubby stick—for my lips and cheeks.

TOM FORD LIPSTICKS: I love all of his lipsticks—from the deep purple of Black Orchid to the autumnal brick red of Deep Mink—for their rich consistency and vibrant pigments. They never dry your lips or bleed beyond the pucker line. And the packaging is insanely chic, of course.

SKYN ICELAND EYE GELS: I never get dressed for an event without applying these patches first. They have a cooling effect and dissolve any puffiness. Wear them for ten minutes and you'll look like you slept for an extra hour. Fashion Week essential!

ARMANI LUMINOUS SILK FOUNDATION: Ask any makeup artist to name a favorite product and this liquid magic will top the list. It is soft and light on your skin and you don't need much of it for great coverage.

TARTE MASCARA: It drives me crazy when a mascara becomes dry and clumpy within a week of use. Tarte's Lights, Camera, Lashes formula has conditioning ingredients, so it always feels soft and looks natural. For those tiny inner and lower lashes, I also use Givenchy Phenom, which has an ingenious ball-shaped applicator.

ARCONA TRIAD PADS: The scent of these cranberry toner pads instantly makes me happy. They cleanse away makeup, tone, and hydrate skin with antioxidants, too. I never travel without them—they're a lifesaver on a long flight.

SMASHBOX LIMITLESS LIQUID LINER PEN: For me, it's all about precision. I love this pen applicator, because you can hold it and draw a line with a steady hand. It doesn't move or run or clump. Plus, it's waterproof.

ZOYA NAIL POLISH IN RILEY: This is the perfect deep Bordeaux for a high-impact manicure. It's my must-have shade for fall and winter. I discovered this line of toxin-free polishes when I was pregnant and now I'm a forever fan.

Of course, these are *my* personal heroes. They work with my lifestyle and complement my features. To find your own lifesaving products, go to makeup counters and experiment, read up on the runway trends every season, and check out beauty blogs. I stay on top of what's hot by contributing to *The Zoe Report,* my daily newsletter, and reading fashion magazines every month.

HANDS ON

Manicures have become masterpieces, with all the new nail art and creative techniques out there. Personally, I tend to play it pretty straightforward, but you will never catch me with chipped or peeling polish. I talk with my hands a lot, so my nails are always front and center. When I don't have time for a professional manicure, I make sure to take a moment to do my own. My preferences in polish go in two distinct directions: a clean, pinkish nude or rich, sumptuous Bordeaux.

I've learned some simple ways to extend a mani or pedi a few extra days, though. First, always use your own polish. Salons sometimes add thinner to make a bottle last longer, but the polish becomes less resilient. This way, you can quickly touch up at home if you get any chips. Also, be sure to polish the tip of the nail with both your color and topcoat to prevent chips. This step alone can double the life of a manicure or pedicure.

Believe it or not, it takes about twelve hours for nails to completely dry. Avoid washing your hands with hot water or even blowing on your nails. Though the latter seems instinctive, warm breath stalls the process. I know sitting idly can be frustrating, but try to take a few minutes to let your nails dry initially, and then before you leave the salon, apply oil to avoid surface smudges. A little later you can run them under cold water to set.

BRUSH UP

When it comes to application, the right brushes are essential—and must be washed with brush cleaner or a mild shampoo every couple of weeks. I have a weakness for Tom Ford's line of brushes, because the white bristles are so soft and dense, but there are many options out there. I rely on five essentials, day to day.

SHADING BRUSH:
With its angled tip and long handle, this brush is perfect for highlighting cheekbones or brow bones with a swath of shimmer.

BRONZER BRUSH:
Ideal for applying loose or compact powder; use it in a circular motion to evenly distribute mineral foundation or bronzer.

CHEEK BRUSH:
I like a slightly rounded brush head with very soft bristles and long, tapered handle to hit the entire apple of my cheek with color.

EYE SHADOW BRUSH:
Use its small, slightly rounded tip for expertly tucking eye shadow into the crease, shading the lids, and sweeping color onto the brow bone.

EYE SHADOW BLEND BRUSH:
Never underestimate the power of blending. I love this brush's ability to diffuse eye shadow color and soften the line of a smoky eye.

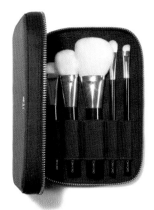

Makeup brushes by Tom Ford

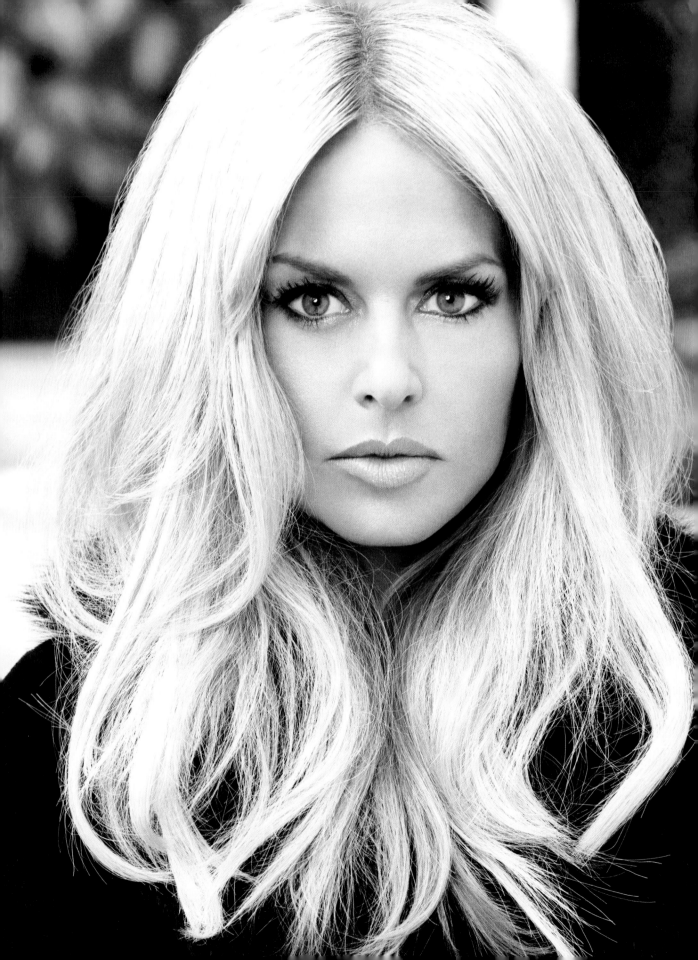

MANE ATTRACTION

My hair has been at my shoulders or longer for as long as I can remember. And as much as I adore the look of a gamine pixie cut and its easy maintenance, I doubt that I will ever go short. Personally, I like the infinite options that come with length, as well as the ability to hide behind a curtain of hair. But in order to preserve these long locks, I'm very keen on maintenance.

Like most women, I adore a professional blowout. Having shiny, silky hair that you can flip over your shoulder is as empowering as a new pair of shoes or a great handbag. Just last year, I partnered with a friend to open DreamDry, a New York salon that offers blowouts and hair styling until 10:00 p.m. every night. (Tell me, who has time to see a hairdresser before sunset during the week?) And while I must admit that I'm an amateur when it comes to blow-drying my own hair, I have learned a few tips and secrets from our stylists. First of all, you shouldn't attempt to blow-dry super wet hair. Have you ever noticed how your hairdresser spends a good ten minutes "predrying" your hair before he or she starts the process? That's because moisture plus heat equals frizz. Let your hair air dry or add low heat with a blow-dryer to get your mane about seventy-five percent dry before you really start styling.

Next, divide hair into multiple three- or four-inch sections. Start with the hair on the crown or around the face—that's what people see first, after all. And if you're like me, your arm is going to start aching soon! Using a round brush, pull the hair taut and aim the nozzle downward on top of the hair to seal the shaft and create shine. Repeat on each section.

Finally, mist your fingers with a holding spray that adds shine and then gently tousle your sleek mane. You can also gently run your palms around your part to flatten flyaways with the residual product.

It's always hard for me to wash my hair after a great blowout. I just want it to last forever—I prolong it as long as four days. I wash my hair only once or twice a week, and many stylists have told me that my mane is amazingly healthy as a result of that habit. You can get away with it if your hair tends to be dry like mine; or you can extend time between washing like I do by adding a little dry shampoo to your roots. It may sound crazy, but women washed their hair once a month back at the turn of the century. That's a long time between shampoos!

I rotate my shampoo and conditioner every month or so in order to avoid buildup. And as someone who colors her hair, I occasionally use a clarifying shampoo to strip away natural buildup from the environment. Chemical and color treatments like straightening or highlighting make hair very porous and absorbent. Every Sunday night, I do a deep conditioning treatment while I watch TV or answer e-mails. When I go to bed, I use a clip to coil it up in a topknot instead of leaving it down. Why? The oils in your hair, not to mention the product buildup from shampoos and serums, can irritate your face and cause breakouts.

While I recommend experimenting to find your favorite products, these are my current ones for healthy hair.

KÉRASTASE CRISTALLISTE SHAMPOO AND CONDITIONER: This line is specially formulated for fine, lengthy hair, which is my exact match. It reduces frizz and makes my hair incredibly shiny.

BYRON WILLIAMS SPIRULINA HAIR SPRAY: I love that this holding spray is certified organic and contains blue algae, which prevents damage and strengthens hair. I use it on flyaways or a topknot to make hair stay put.

GLOSS MODERNE HIGH-GLOSS MASQUE: When my hair needs a spa day, I slather on this treatment to restore its natural luster and hydrate. It can be a lifesaver if you use a lot of heat on your hair with flat irons, curling irons, or blow-dryers.

ORIBE DRY TEXTURIZING SPRAY: I can extend a blowout by three days with this dry hair spray that absorbs oil at the roots and adds body. Keep it in your office for instant day-to-night volume.

HAMADI ORGANICS HEALING SERUM: Scented with ylang-ylang and bergamot, this moisturizing spray treatment for dry, overprocessed tresses refreshes dry ends and leaves my hair incredibly soft. I spritz my entire mane and then comb through to the ends at least twice a week.

PHYLIA CONNECT LEAVE-IN TREATMENT: This spray-on blend of organic ingredients treats both the hair and the scalp. I use it right out of the shower and it lifts my hair at the roots and makes my hair look twice as thick.

ADIR ABERGEL'S THREE STEPS TO AMAZING HAIR

Rachel and I collaborate often on looks for her clients. We have similar beauty sensibilities—we never want a woman to look "done"; rather, she should always exude a fluid, effortless look. To achieve that, we focus first on volume. To get the body that makes hair look so healthy and full, always use a volumizing product on your roots before you start styling. You will see a boost right away. You should invest in a backcomb, which creates height that lasts all day. The secret here is to take very small sections and gently tease or compact the hair at the root before styling.

Next, you need movement. Spray on dry shampoo, even if you just washed your hair. It sounds crazy, but it's a red-carpet secret. This step creates texture, which is the key to movement. During a blow-dry, be sure to let the round brush cool down for about twenty to thirty seconds before you remove it from your hair. That way, you will get some long-lasting bounce.

Finally, shine is a must. It truly makes hair look youthful. Do a weekly deep masque, which will pay off with amazing shine. When you blow-dry your hair, be certain that you flatten the cuticle by using a boar bristle round brush and aiming the nozzle downward. A flat cuticle really reflects light. ■

TOOL TIME

Obviously, we all have different hair profiles and needs when it comes to styling. But there are a few basic tools that will always come in handy for the health and manageability of your mane.

ROUND BRUSHES:
I like a small one-inch boar bristle version for my bangs and a larger one, about three inches in diameter, for the rest of my hair. Natural bristles make your hair much shinier.

POWERFUL HAIR DRYER WITH ACCESSORIES:
More wattage can cut your blow-dry time in half, so look for those with no fewer than 1300 watts. Right now, I'm using Sultra's 1650-watt powerful ionic dryer, which does the job fast and makes my hair glossy. A good diffuser is essential if you have curly or wavy hair—it helps to prevent frizz by minimizing the intensity of the airflow. A nozzle, which always comes with a dryer, will direct the air and prevent hair from burning.

WIDE-TOOTHED COMB:
Hairstylists always say "Never brush wet hair,' because it will cause breakage. Instead, I use a wide-toothed comb right out of the shower.

MINI FLAT IRON:
Personally, I avoid using too much direct heat on my hair, because I don't trust my hand. But I do like the miniature version for taming flyaways or getting a kink out of my bangs. Flat ironing is a good way to achieve a super-sleek look.

CURLING IRON OR ROLLERS:
For achieving sexy beach waves or adding some volume to the crown of your hair, a curling iron or wand with a one-inch barrel or hot rollers will come in handy.

CLEAR ELASTICS:
Sometimes you just don't have those extra twenty minutes to style your hair. For that reason, I think a few handy clear elastics are as essential as a blow-dryer. Ponytails, braids, a half updo—the possibilities are endless!

Left: Jerry Hall. Right: Kate Moss.

ICONIC BEAUTY LOOKS

Trends come and go, but there are a handful of hair and makeup effects that never swerve out of style. When in doubt, try one of these looks with staying power.

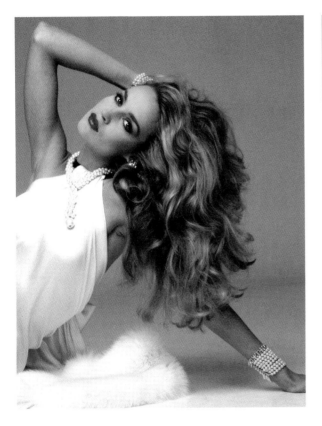

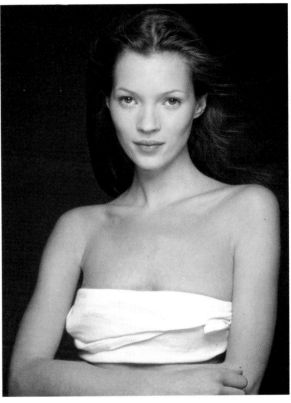

RED LIPS

Love it: Every woman must wear bombshell red lipstick for one day in her life, at least. It's the pinnacle of glamour.

Get it: Experiment with undertones such as blues or corals to find your most flattering shade. And be sure to shape lips with a nude pencil first to keep the bold color in place.

GLOWING SKIN

Love it: Who doesn't want to radiate health and natural beauty? It makes you so approachable.

Get it: Moisturize your skin and then add just a touch of concealer beneath the eyes. Finish with a light bronzing powder that has a hint of shimmer.

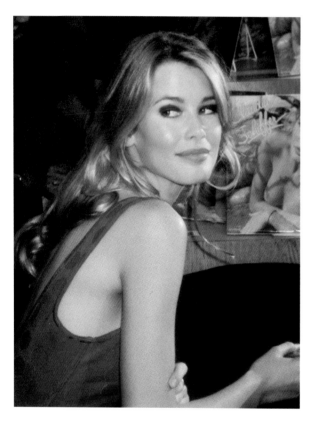

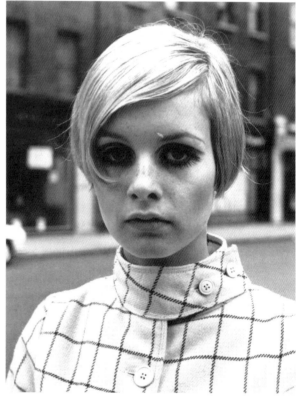

THE SMOKY EYE

Love it: There is no trick I love more for transforming a look from day to night. Your eyes instantly become the focal point of your face.

Get it: I like to see variations on the traditional black liner. Experiment with colors like a slate blue or olive green. Even a rich mocha brown can stand out as much as black. Trace your top lash line with liquid liner and then dot liner between the lower lashes. Immediately begin smudging the lines for a soft, smoky effect. Then, brush the upper lid with a shadow and blend the color right to the line above the upper lashes.

MAJOR LASHES

Love it: This sixties-inspired look reads ultra modern and allows you to go full force with a dramatic lip in any hue.

Get it: Whether it's with a few coats of mascara or faux lashes, be sure to hit the lower lash line, too. You can also curl your lashes for more drama. I like to add individual fake lashes just to the upper outer corners for an extra upward kick.

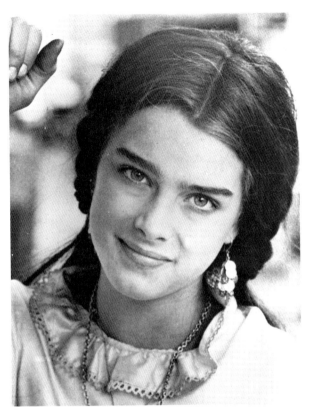

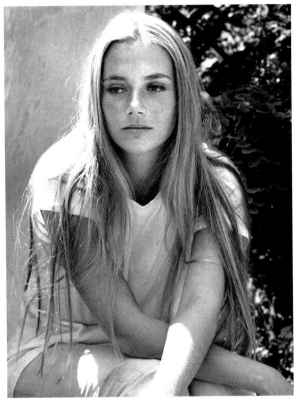

STATEMENT BROW

Love it: A full brow can alter the whole composition of your face and gives you options on how to define them, from thick arches to strong arrows. I once overplucked my own brows, so now I tweeze them rarely and very carefully. If yours tend to grow thick and unruly, plan to groom them monthly.

Get it: You can always bolster your brow with a pencil or an angled brush and powder. Or, gently brush naturally dark hairs upward and outward and then set with a clear brow gel before shaping.

STICK-STRAIGHT HAIR

Love it: I love that this classic style can feel retro or modern, depending on the rest of your look. It also brings all the attention to your neck and face.

Get it: Whether you blow it out yourself or visit a salon, don't forget to finish with a shine serum to prevent flyaways and create depth.

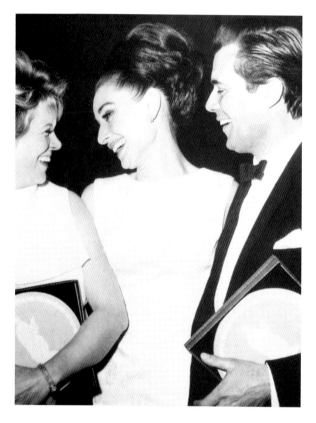

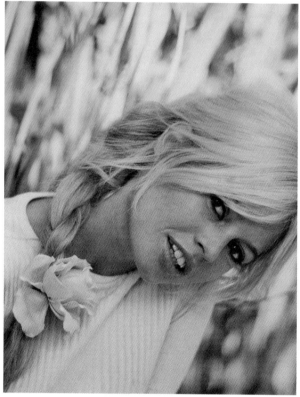

TOPKNOT

Love it: The young girls in my office are fanatics of this chic high bun, and vary it by incorporating a French braid or even a cool clip.

Get it: I like the old-school method of coiling a high ponytail and securing it with pins. To make it more free spirited, I pull some tendrils around my face and grab a few ends out of the knot so it appears a little undone.

BRAID

Love it: I've been obsessed with braids ever since I was a little girl. A braided updo manages to look both youthful and sophisticated at the same time.

Get it: Whether it's a fishtail, French, or the milkmaid style across your crown, this will become your new favorite look, I swear.

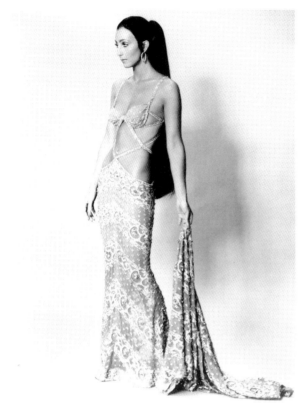

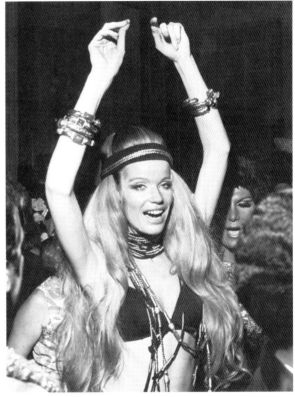

PONYTAIL

Love it: Never mind the fact that pulling your hair off your face gives you an instant facelift—there is something so sleek about a ponytail.

Get it: Experiment with the possibilities, from a high one with lots of volume and movement to a low pony with a center part and a pin-straight tail.

BEACH WAVES

Love it: A cascade of textured waves that frames the face always looks effortlessly sensual. The look works equally well with a bathing suit and ball gown. Sometimes I go to sleep with my damp hair in a few braids in order to get those sexy ripples.

Get it: Thankfully, you don't need to live by an ocean to get these waves. There are texturizing products galore that make your hair look like you just went for a swim—many of them are even called "beach waves." To get the look with a curling iron, be sure to vary the direction of the waves you create so it doesn't look too uniform. You want the end result to be windswept and a little messy, which you can achieve by bending over and flipping your hair a few times.

THE WHITE HOUSE

It took me years to come to appreciate my parents' amazing taste. Growing up, I didn't think of them as design savvy and forward thinking. In fact, I considered them eccentric and kind of weird. We lived in a suburb of Manhattan and the prevailing décor in my neighborhood was anything but contemporary and sleek. Most of my friends' houses featured traditional French or colonial furniture sets, wing chairs, heavy floral drapery, and lots of oriental rugs. Our house, however, could have been described as a stark tribute to streamlined, midcentury modern design.

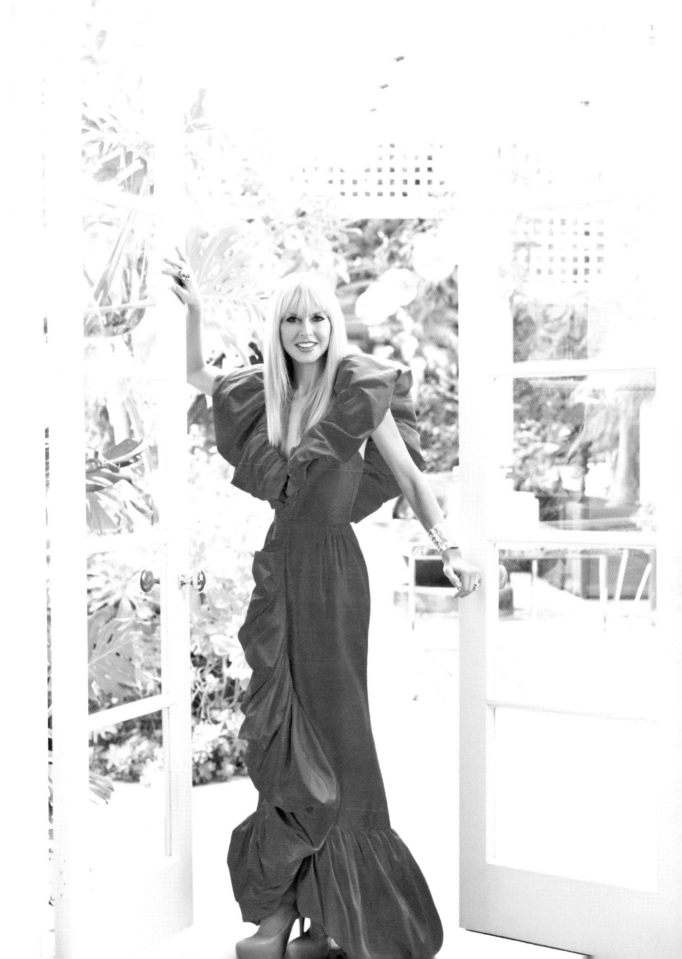

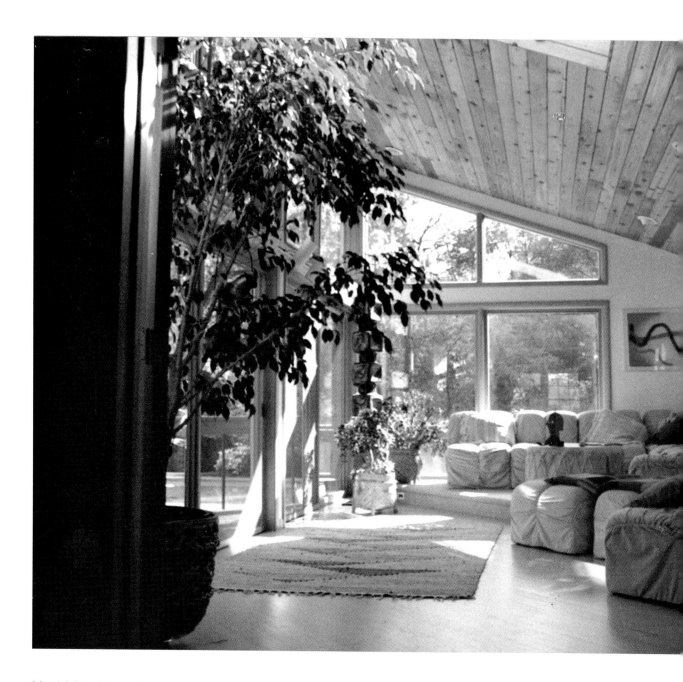

*My childhood home in
Short Hills, New Jersey*

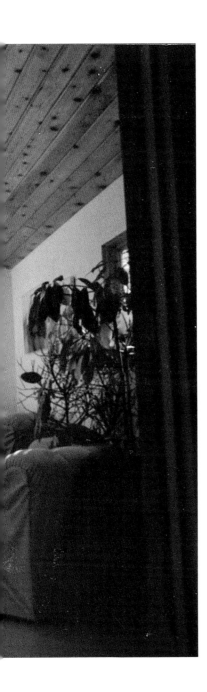

The entire interior was neutral, including our walls, B&B Italia sofa, and natural fiber rugs. My dad relaxed and read the *New York Times* in a cognac-colored Eames leather recliner with a matching ottoman, but most of the other pieces fell into a muted palette of ecru, linen, and blond wood. Then, there was the art. Our neighbors favored glossy oil paintings in ornate gilt frames. Hunt scenes, portraits, ships at sea—that kind of thing. The Rosenzweig house? Photo collages layered with aggressive text by Barbara Kruger, graphic political prints that commented on apartheid by Keith Haring, and disquieting paintings by modern realist Mark Tansey. My parents followed the art scene closely and collected pieces by the most talented up-and-comers—my dad will elaborate on how to start collecting art on page 166. It all seems so cool now, but back then I wondered why we couldn't hang just one watercolor of flowers.

Even my bedroom was a study in clean aestheticism. It, too, was entirely neutral with a big white trundle bed in the corner, except, of course, for my own art: bright Technicolor posters of boys—the likes of Erik Estrada and Shaun Cassidy—graced my walls until I was eight. Later, Duran Duran and George Michael were my crushes du jour. I think I became boy crazy before I could even talk! My focus centered on my bedroom closet even then. Let's just say there was never enough room for all my thrift store finds and accessories. And much like today, I organized my clothes and shoes according to color. Truth be told, my school outfits were more of a priority than my homework. Shocking, right?

In my junior year of college at George Washington University in D.C., I met Rodger. He was a waiter at a restaurant where I started working as a hostess; we became inseparable after our first date. (Much more on that magical night in Chapter 6.) As soon as I graduated, we both moved to New York. My first apartment was a thousand-square-foot studio that I decorated with stray hand-me-downs from my parents and pieces like shag rugs and lamps I found at flea markets. Working nonstop, I didn't put too much time or thought into my décor. All my energy went toward my career—and my clothes. When Rodger and I moved in together, we never really established a home. We relocated every two years to better rentals, because that's what New Yorkers do. I distinctly remember going through my "shabby chic" phase at our place on Thirty-fifth and Park with its overstuffed country French chairs and distressed furniture. It was beautiful and trendy, but it never felt like a reflection of me. I would walk into my apartment and, quite honestly, feel a bit uncomfortable. I realized that if my home didn't embrace my true aesthetic, I would always feel like a guest.

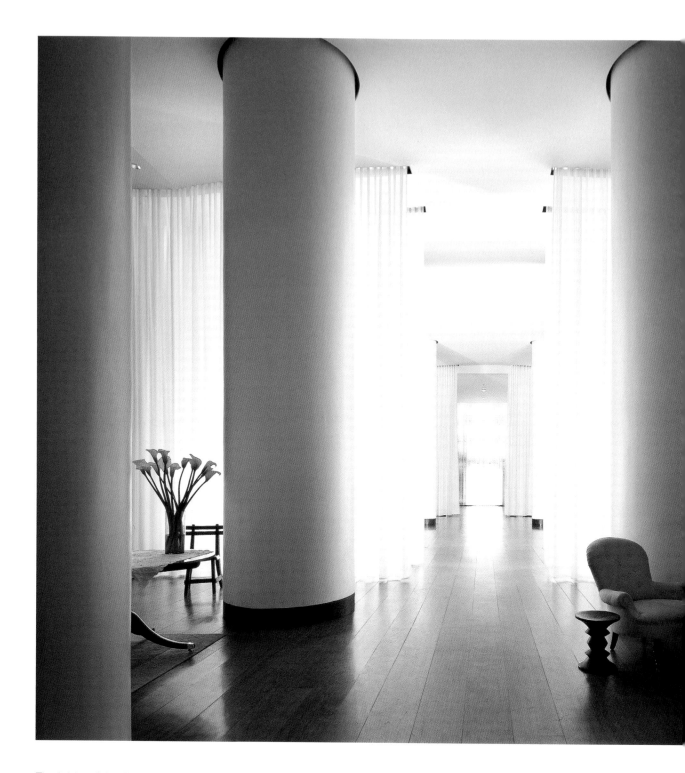

*The lobby of the Delano
Hotel, Miami*

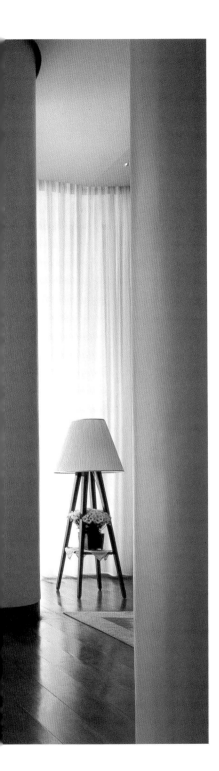

At that point, though, I hadn't yet figured out my own design sense. Thankfully, a visit to the Delano Hotel in Miami's South Beach when it first opened helped me solve that dilemma. The lobby, designed by Philippe Starck and conceived as an indoor-outdoor space, was an airy haven of little enclaves separated by sheer white curtains that led out to the pool. The natural light alone made it feel like a beautiful beach with blond hardwood floors and scattered cabanas. The lobby instantly brought me back to our family vacations to the South of France. Statement pieces by Starck and Marc Newson and art by Man Ray added distinction. It was my idea of heaven. I looked at Rodger and said, "I want our home to be like this…for-ev-er."

Once we returned to New York, we even brought in a decorator—Delphine Krakoff—to transform our loft on Ninety-fifth Street into an East Coast urban facsimile of the Delano. Too bad it was just a rental.

When we moved to Los Angeles in December 2002, my clean and contemporary design sense was right on the mark. Midcentury modern houses beckoned with their uniform lines and floor-to-ceiling glass windows. I could finally rely on bright natural light instead of lamps and fixtures. Thankfully, the furniture we already had suited the architecture of our first house. Especially since Rodger and I had carted so much of it—from an Arco lamp to a Philippe Starck sofa to a Christian Liaigre bench—across the country. Each of those pieces, except for the Arco lamp, which broke during the move, is still in our current house in Beverly Hills.

And now, decades later, the midcentury ranch I thought was so odd as a kid is a muse. That sparse and modern aesthetic my parents always embraced appeals to me on so many levels. Our first big investments were a neutral B&B Italia sofa and an Eames lounger in white leather that I bought for Rodger. Maybe our son will look around one day and think we're a bit weird, too. That's just fine.

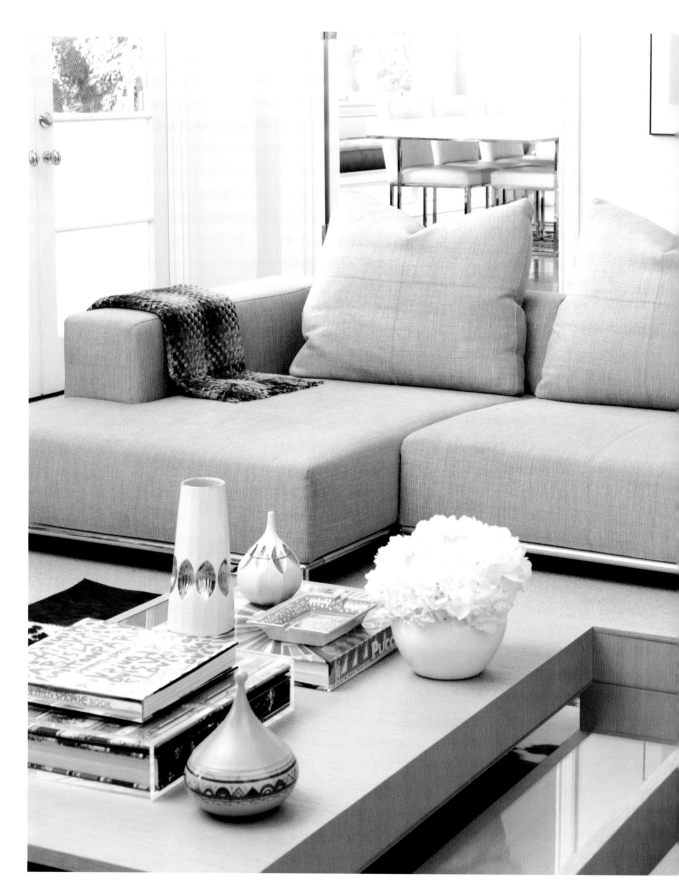

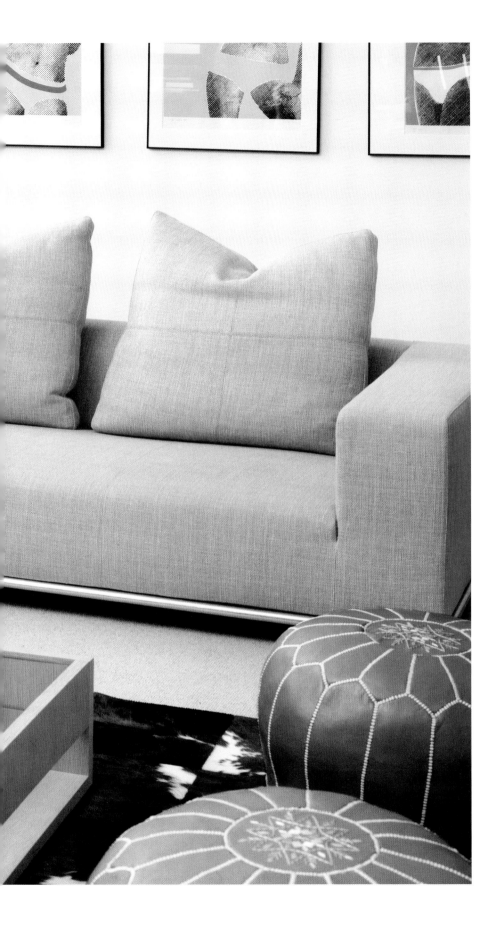

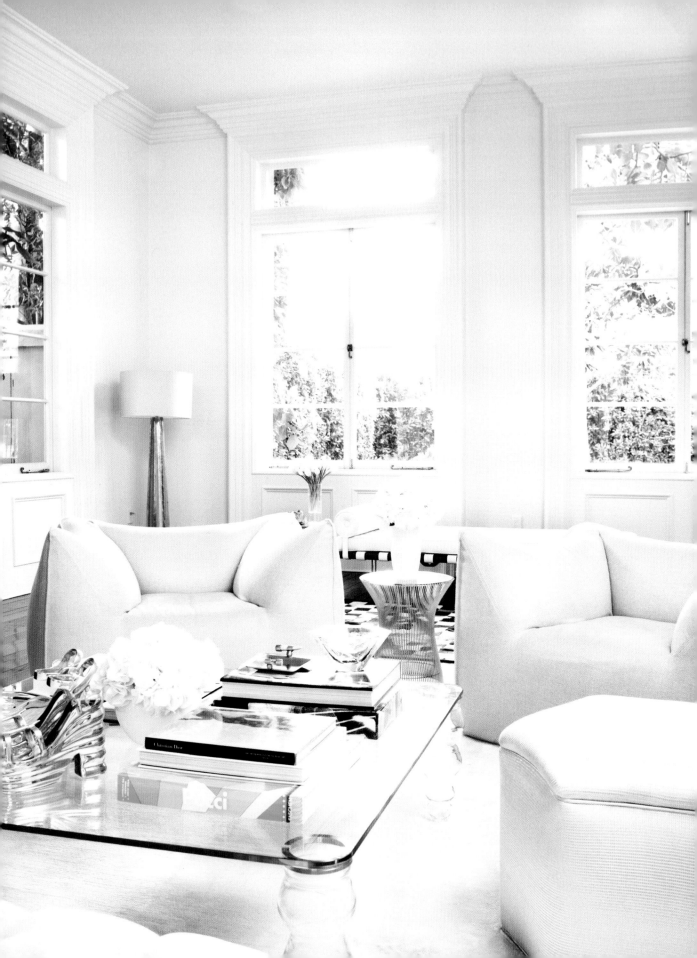

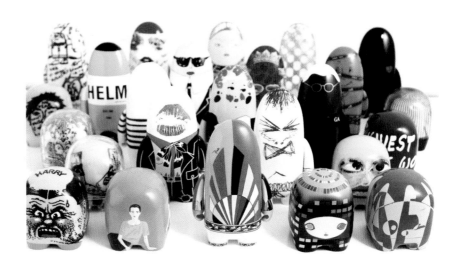

PASSION AS INSPIRATION

Decorating a home—or even a room—requires confidence and vision.
To me, it's a lot like the process of putting together an outfit. You're using
different elements to create one overall, cohesive look. Of course, furniture and rugs and window treatments often require much more financial
output than earrings or a pair of skinny jeans. But if you focus on your
personal style and your passions, you already have a jump on how to
create a setting.

> "DECORATING A HOME—OR EVEN A ROOM—REQUIRES
> CONFIDENCE AND VISION. TO ME, IT'S A LOT LIKE
> THE PROCESS OF PUTTING TOGETHER AN OUTFIT."

Clearly, my first love has always been fashion. My dad likes to say
"Fashion is Rachel's art." He's right. Almost every accent in our house
relates to my obsession. A collection of Visionaire vinyl dolls by Kidrobot—
from a mini Karl Lagerfeld to a tiny Vivienne Westwood—all speak to my
worship of and respect for my favorite fashion icons. On my coffee table
in the living room, a pair of silver-plated shoes sits atop a stack of fashion
books. These fashion tomes, by the way, make great statement pieces
on a table or mantel. Plus, guests can flip through them during a cocktail
party. It's no surprise to me that so many museums around the world, from
the Met in New York to the Grand Trianon at Versailles, have exhibited

fashion as conceptual art. When I was in my twenties in New York, I hung vintage flapper dresses on my apartment walls and displayed a Versace chainmail dress on a coffee table. It still seems silly to stash all my fabulous pieces in a dark closet. I want to see my "art" and be inspired by it throughout the day.

Now, I surround myself with fashion photographs and prints. In the master bedroom, an entire wall is covered by a dozen art deco antique Hermès ads from the 1920s and 1930s. Right now, I'm coveting the 1963 "Bubble" series of models suspended in giant plastic balls above the River Seine in Paris by Melvin Sokolsky. His black-and-white photographs are absolutely breathtaking both in their composition and design.

"MY CLOSET IS MY IDEA OF A FANTASTIC MUSEUM."

As much as I love accessories, you won't find random knickknacks in my house. However, people who know me well have noticed my array of designer ceramic trinket trays and vibrant ashtrays by the likes of Hermès, Gucci, and Bulgari. In fact, my collection continues to expand, thanks to thoughtful contributions from friends and family. They look stunning all grouped together or scattered throughout the house. If you find a particular object that speaks to you, such as vintage decanters or Murano glass pieces, start amassing and make them the centerpiece of a table or shelves.

My closet is my idea of a fantastic museum. Sometimes, I artfully arrange my clutches on shelves so I can step back and admire them like Rembrandts. Printed silk scarves, especially designer vintage ones, look so chic and add a splash of color to a wall in any room. You can either iron one and mat it yourself or have a professional framer handle the job. I love to see a scattering of shoes on bookshelves or an étagère. A pair of vintage Ferragamo wedges used as bookends? Adorable! Another great nod to fashion is a vintage dress form, which you can buy online for under a hundred dollars. It becomes a colorful and textural sculpture when you add a fantastic piece like a vintage Pucci dress to it, or an architectural Thierry Mugler gown. It's art you can refresh or change out as often as you like.

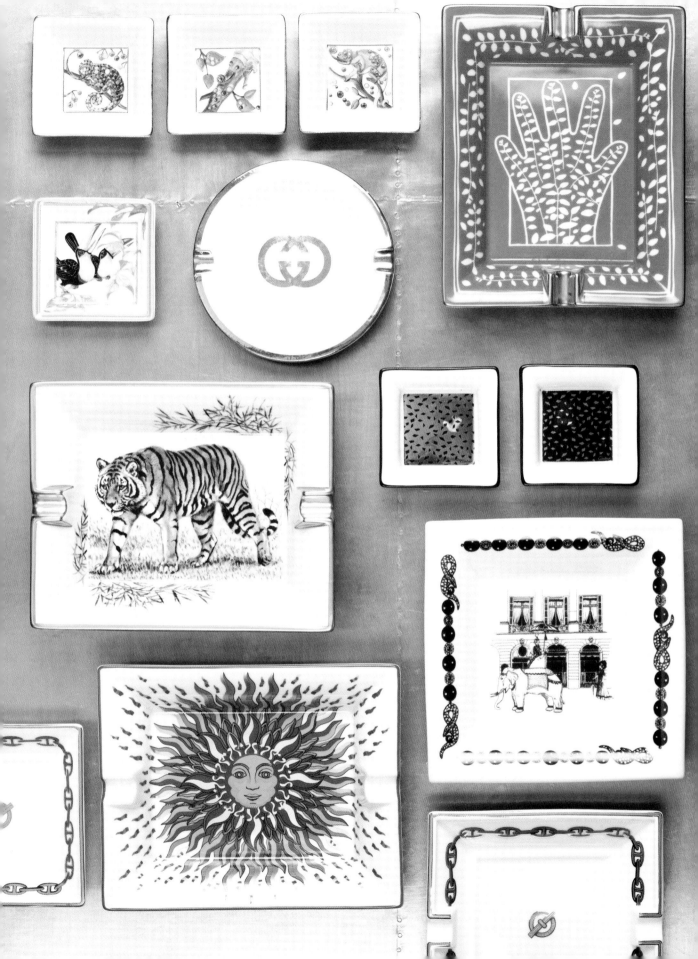

RON ROSENZWEIG ON BUYING ART

As Rachel mentioned, Leslie and I have been collecting art since the 1960s. Sometimes we buy a major painting to celebrate our anniversary, such as the Frank Stella we acquired to celebrate ten years together. It's a true passion.

If you're looking to start collecting, first of all, buy what you love. We didn't even realize that art could be an investment when we purchased our first pieces, which were African sculptures and American Indian art; we were just drawn to the works. Later, we realized that we both had a passion for abstract modern artists and so we started educating ourselves.

It's important to learn about different periods—you never know whom or what you might discover along the way. I think it's a good idea to sub-scribe to art magazines to see as much as you can. Early on, Leslie and I would go to different galleries in Soho to get a sense of the landscape; she even took contemporary art classes at a local museum. Another great way to expand your knowledge—and collection—is to meet other people looking to buy art. In the early eighties, we joined a group affiliated with the New Museum in New York and we all shared information on new artist studios and exhibits. Galleries, art walks, and the young patron programs at museums are great places to socialize, too.

Once you purchase your first major piece, make it the centerpiece of your décor. What we have found over the years is that rather than buy something to match the palette or style of the room, we let the art become the focal point. A painting can bring a whole space together with its size, colors, and tone. ■

COMMIT, INVEST, REJOICE

Decorating can be daunting, because interior design is all about com-mitment. Big-ticket items like couches and dining room tables require a lot of consideration. Before we bought the B&B Italia sofa that is now in our family room, Rodger and I visited it in the showroom and discussed it countless times. The same goes for our Philippe Starck marble-topped table and white couch.

Before settling on a large piece that will greatly affect your surroundings, I suggest that you contemplate the purchase just as you would an expensive designer handbag or coat. I ask myself a few questions before I begin acquiring major furnishings.

CAN I LIVE WITH THE COLOR AND DESIGN FOR A DECADE?

I always opt for neutral, because we can accessorize with color in throws and cushions. On the other hand, you might crave colorful major furnishings and temper the overall palette with muted accents. In deciding on the design, we tend to invest in well-crafted pieces with timeless modern design instead of on-trend furniture. Pieces that boast "great bones" retain their value and last a lifetime.

HOW DOES IT WORK WITH MY OTHER PIECES?
Take a picture of the piece in question and then take it home and look at in the context of your space. You don't want to invest in a major item that might force you to redo your entire interior to make it flow well.

IS IT A SHOW PONY OR A USABLE PIECE?
I have been to homes in which certain furniture is completely off-limits. Maybe it's an original Hans Wegner chair or a spindly antique side table that's unsteady. My personal feeling on "don't touch" pieces is that they can intimidate your guests. You always want to make sure your furniture makes people feel comfortable.

WILL I HAVE A STROKE OVER A STAIN?
As someone with mostly white décor, I have learned to pray and look the other way when a guest sips red wine while sitting on my tufted white Chesterfield couch. You can only be so vigilant, right? Be sure you have such investment pieces pretreated for any spills. Legend has it that Coco Chanel let only certain visitors sit on her neutral suede couch!

DO I ABSOLUTELY LOVE, LOVE, LOVE IT?
It's my go-to rule whenever I buy something valuable. I usually ask myself if I would be absolutely heartbroken if I didn't take it home. Sometimes, I even wait a week before purchasing to see if I am truly obsessed or just infatuated.

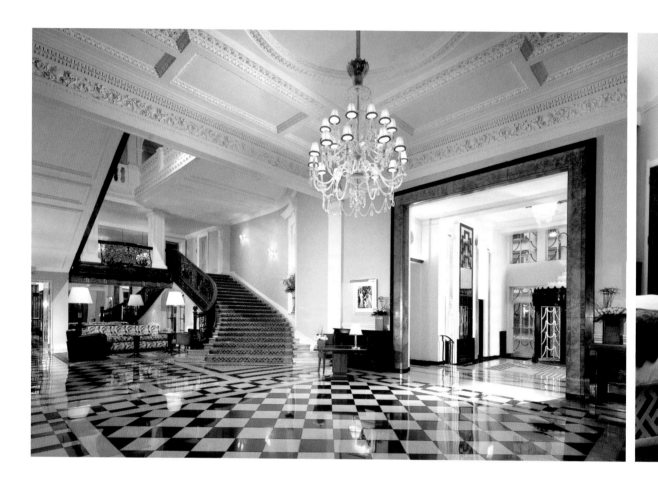

Left to right: The lobby of the Claridge's Hotel, London. Suites at the Claridge's Hotel, London.

MY INSPIRATIONS

Gorgeous hotels and restaurants can make excellent sources for décor ideas, because they're designed to be both elegant and inviting. So much thought is funneled into every detail, from the comfort and configuration of the seating to the placement of simple accents. If you visit a fantastic location—whether it's a cool café or a chic private home—be sure to take notes. Throughout the years, I have found a few favorite places to stay, dine, visit, and glean ideas.

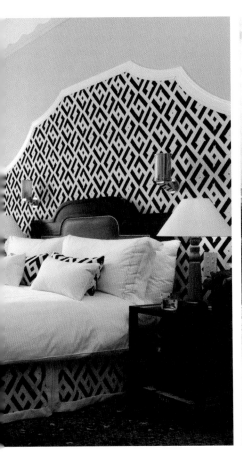

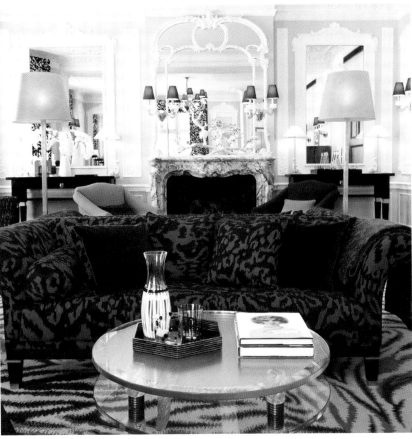

CLARIDGE'S HOTEL LOBBY AND SUITES: This art deco setting manages to marry masculine and feminine to stunning effect. The lobby features a black-and-white checkerboard floor with leather club chairs and a graceful ornate crystal chandelier by Dale Chihuly. Each suite feels decidedly different, but shares a few hallmarks of deco design like geometric mirrors and piped furniture. Your house can be eclectic from room to room, too. Rather than try to extend an overall theme throughout, infuse each area with its own personality and carry over one element, like a color or a chevron print.

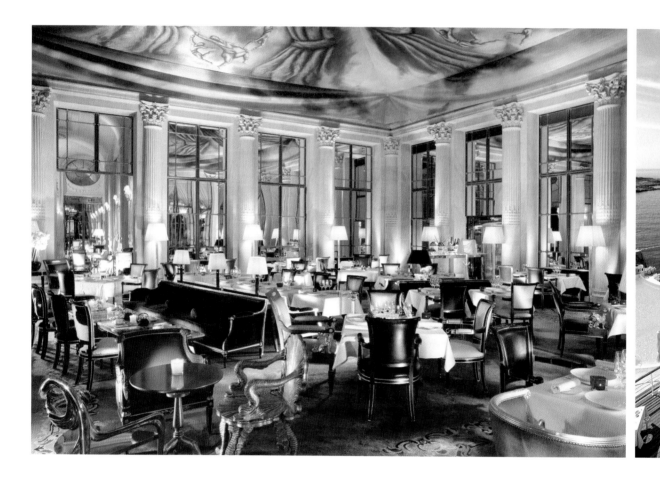

RESTAURANT LE DALÍ AT LE MEURICE: Philippe Starck oversaw the design of this gorgeous eatery with its mismatched bergère chairs, Doric columns, and whimsical touches like a lamp with drawers and seating with ladies' shoes as legs. A dining table with an assortment of chairs always looks unique and more eye-catching, in my opinion. And the best part is that you can nab a collection of different styles at a flea market. I also appreciate the bold statement that a suede or velvet banquette in a smoky gray or pale mink brown makes as seating at the table.

HOTEL DU CAP: Built originally as a private mansion for writers, this château-style hotel perched on the coast of the French Riviera has become an outpost for actors, designers, and artists. But it's the twenty-two acres of towering pines, tropical gardens, topiaries, and the saltwater infinity pool that make me gasp whenever I visit. People say that Marc Chagall sketched the impressive view from one of the cabanas back in the 1960s. Think of your backyard as a giant living room and set up little pockets of

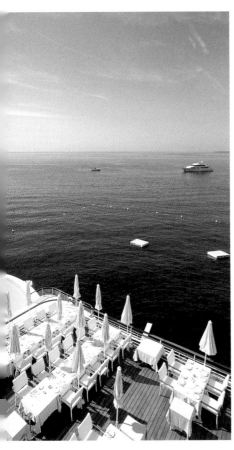

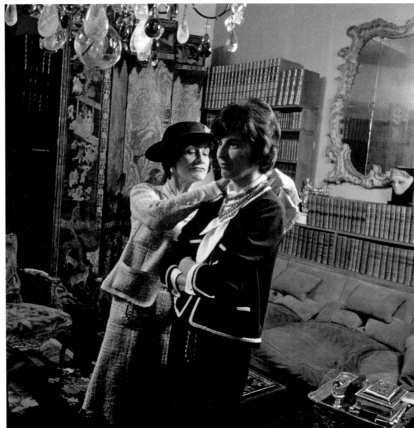

inviting furniture. You can use chaise lounges, overstuffed outdoor cushions, and even colorful towels. We set up a dining table beneath an arbor in our back space and occasionally dine al fresco on warm nights.

COCO CHANEL'S PARIS APARTMENT: When I had the honor of visiting Coco Chanel's apartment at 31 rue Cambon (it's closed to the public!) I didn't know where to look first. From the interlocking Cs chandelier to the mirrored spiral staircase to the huge Chinese screens etched with camellias, every inch of this four-room flat above the original Chanel boutique is impossibly ornate and elegant. Believe it or not, she only entertained here—she had a suite at the Ritz, where she slept most nights. I love that as a Leo, Chanel adorned her space with lions. Picking a motif meaningful to you makes it much easier to choose small treasures for display. If you favor a certain animal, flower, or even decade, look for interesting pieces that express your particular taste.

COMMUNAL CHEER

The rooms where people gather become the most beloved and most frequently used. It may be the kitchen, where a few friends chat at the table while you make scones, or a family room that plays host to the bustling kids' dinner table every Thanksgiving. In my house, these two, along with the living and dining areas, must be warm, stylish, and functional.

TO LOOK OVER AND SEE MY TWO FAVORITE GUYS
WITH BEDHEAD SLEEPILY WATCHING ME MAKE
OATMEAL OR TOAST BAGELS MAKES ME SO HAPPY."

In the living room—which we originally deemed the "white room"—a giant sofa languishes across from a set of deep, cozy Mario Bellini chairs. A console with two vintage French blown-glass lamps that feature black-and-white shades lend a little Parisian flair to the space. I think our guests have always been a little leery of tracking in wet leaves or accidentally spilling coffee on the white silk rug—I wanted the space to feel more welcoming. To do that, I turned one corner into a parking lot for Skyler's vintage toy cars and planes and boats. It's funny to spot his playthings in this otherwise pristine space, but it definitely makes the room feel more lived in.

Our family room happens to house quite a few of Skyler's playthings, too. Are you seeing a theme here? In this area off the kitchen, a huge sectional faces a media center and we have a cool little bar space to the left that is strictly Rodger's domain. I swear, I have never gone back there. When friends or family come over to watch a movie or casually hang out, we overtake the sofa and a tufted white Barcelona ottoman and even a few poufs. Leather poufs can serve as a glamourous alternative to additional seating. The whole room is an organic environment for sharing a few glasses of wine or passing around a bowl of popcorn.

But isn't it always the kitchen that becomes the unofficial clubhouse? No matter how many candelabras or bouquets of fresh flowers you put in the dining room, a crowd congregates around wherever the host can be found cooking. I love our eat-in kitchen—I make breakfast for Rodger and Skyler every morning. To look over and see my two favorite guys with bedhead sleepily watching me make oatmeal or toast bagels makes me so happy.

A QUICK PRIMER ON PAINT

Selecting paint colors makes me nervous, because it requires a major leap of faith. In our current home, we had the interior painted a shade of white recommended to us by a dear friend, who happens to be a brilliant designer. But we bought the shade from a different brand of paint than she suggested. Guess what? Every wall ended up a blush color that reminded me of pale pink roses. I felt like I was trapped in a sixteen-year-old girl's bedroom!

What we learned the hard way was simply to do this: Always paint a wide swatch of your wall in a chosen paint color and sit with it for at least twenty-four hours. You want to see the effect during full sunlight *and* at dusk. Personally, I like white only because I view walls as a blank canvas for art and a backdrop for beautiful furniture and accessories. I have dreamed of painting a wall a rich emerald green, but I can't bring myself to deviate from my neutral aesthetic. That's not to say that I don't appreciate a colorful room in another home, of course. I envy people who have the guts to go over the top with a vibrant blue or deep plum in a dining room.

During the aforementioned painting fiasco, I also learned about the different finishes, since they profoundly affect the end result, too. Each of these different types of paint works best in a particular area.

MATTE:
I like the flat, nonreflective look of this finish, which best covers the imperfections of an old house. It works on ceilings and in living rooms or bedrooms. Caveat: Smudges won't clean off with a sponge—you have to touch up spots.

EGGSHELL:
The slightest sheen makes this velvety finish easier to wipe away, but it also marks up easily, so avoid using it in the kitchen or bathrooms.

SATIN:
This finish with a pearl-like sheen works well for bathrooms and kitchens, because it withstands humidity best.

SEMIGLOSS:
All our crown moldings, casings, and doors are painted in this slightly shiny coat that makes trim stand out from walls. I love the slight luster.

GLOSS:
Some people adore the high drama of this seriously shiny paint, which can reflect light like a mirror. Be careful with this one, though: If your walls aren't completely smooth, every blemish will be magnified.

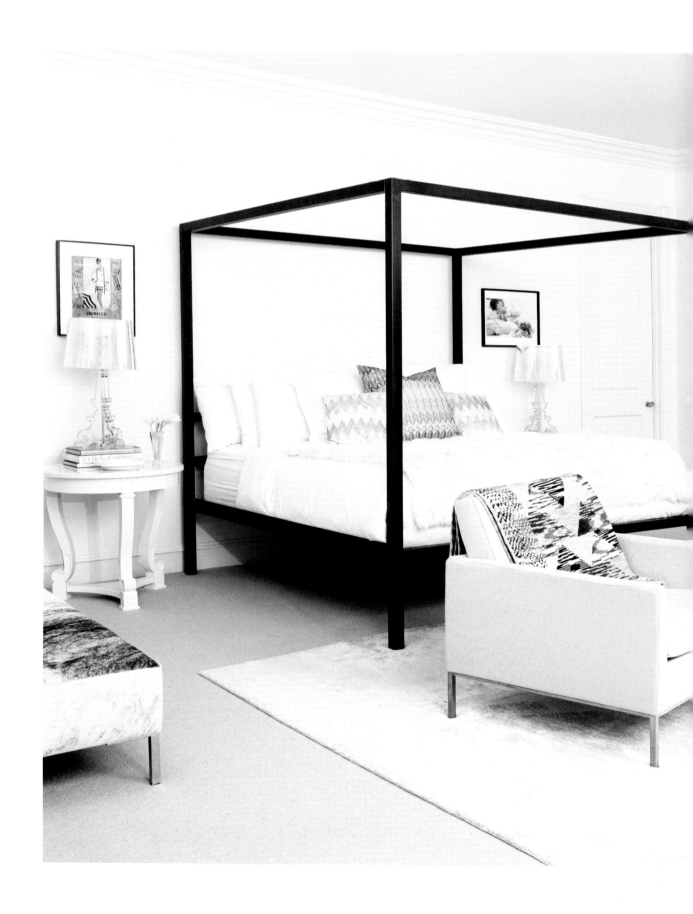

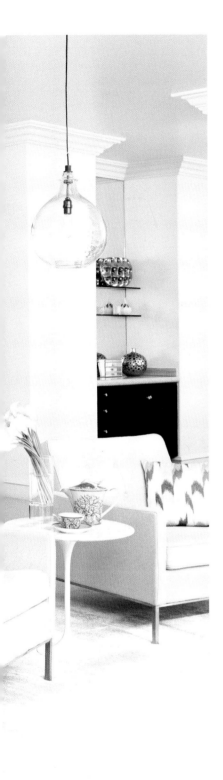

My bedroom

BEDROOM BLISS

A bedroom should be the most serene and comfortable room in your home—a zen area where you emotionally shed the day's hurdles. In past apartments and houses, this room often doubled as a work zone for me. I never intended to do business at the end of the night or first thing in the morning, but invariably I woke up, grabbed my laptop, and started returning e-mails. With technology so mobile today, it's easy to snuggle up next to your phone and check your messages in the middle of the night. Don't do it. Trust me, you don't want to feel anxious or frustrated in bed because of a work situation. That feeling will carry over and affect your sleep. I created a sitting area in my bedroom to ensure that I don't do business between the sheets. A couple of mod club chairs and a small marble end table in front of the fireplace make the perfect configuration for flipping through magazines and sipping a cup of English breakfast tea or taking a fashion emergency call from a client. If your bedroom real estate is limited, a side chair in a corner with a Moroccan pouf can become a viable workspace, too. Add a floor lamp to create a special area to write notes or to make a packing list for an upcoming vacation.

In keeping with my fixation on natural light and an ambient setting, our bed faces a wall of windows with shutters that we rarely close. When we do, there are Lucite lamps on the nightstands and a vintage hanging pendant light above the sitting area that all create a soft hue. I'm a fiend for facing windows from my bed, because I like to see stars and wake up to the sun. But I'm also intrigued by floating a bed in the middle of a room instead of abutting a wall—but try it only if you have enough space to anchor the bed in the center without creating an obstruction.

Some say that the secret to a successful marriage is separate bathrooms. Maybe that's what accounts for Rodger and my twenty-plus years together! We are lucky enough to each have our own private domain off the master bedroom. (We have separate closets, too, which I think may be the *real* secret to a happy marriage.) In my mind, a bathroom should be a serene setting, because it's where you start your day, for the most part. It's the last stop before bed, too. You can make it a more chic and personal setting with beautiful perfume bottles arranged like art pieces and fresh flowers. I display my scents on a mirrored tray, which highlights the curves of each bottle and flacon. A pair of midcentury modern leather cube chairs—plus one miniature version for Skyler—face a mirrored vanity where I do my hair and makeup every morning. I always put away my cosmetics or creams and hair tools. We all work hard in front of the mirror to look effortlessly gorgeous and glamourous. Why leave all the incriminating evidence behind?

Sleep On It

When it comes to linens, I am of two distinct minds. I love the crisp clean look of all white sheets and duvet with a simple border, such as the classic Frette Hotel line. An ivory sheepskin throw strewn at the end of our four-poster mahogany bed makes it cozy, too. But I'm also crazy for the infusion of color a room gets with a vibrant knit Missoni coverlet or chevron throw pillows. My solution? Invest in two different bedding sets that satisfy your different moods. That way, you won't feel so pressured to pick the perfect comforter and sheet set.

Still, choosing colors and prints can be overwhelming. Good bedding is an investment, for sure, as the price of a luxury Egyptian cotton flat sheet can rival the cost of a great pair of sunglasses, though there are great lesser-priced options, too. One way to whittle down choices is to consider possibilities from a fashion perspective. Look in your closet and let your wardrobe help dictate which hues and textures will suit you. If you favor clean lines and unadorned fabrics in clothes, a Versailles-inspired brocade comforter doesn't fit your aesthetic. Do you have a peasant blouse for every day of the week? Look for Moroccan-inspired bedding with Moorish motifs. You want to invest in bedding that you can live with for at least a year or so. I always opt for the more classic, even basic, styles for that very reason.

Designers like Missoni, Diane von Furstenberg, Donna Karan, and Ralph Lauren all offer coordinating sets that reflect their sartorial sense. Ralph Lauren's pieces, as you can imagine, evoke a more equestrian club setting with muted paisleys, while Donna Karan's collection is as minimalist and sleek as her clothes. I dream of designing linens some time soon, because I believe a bed should be a visual and physical sanctuary. Technically, you spend about twenty-five percent of your life in your bed, right? In that case, it should be perfect. My set will most likely embrace my passion for great tailoring with crisp lines, clean stitching, and glamour. Stay tuned.

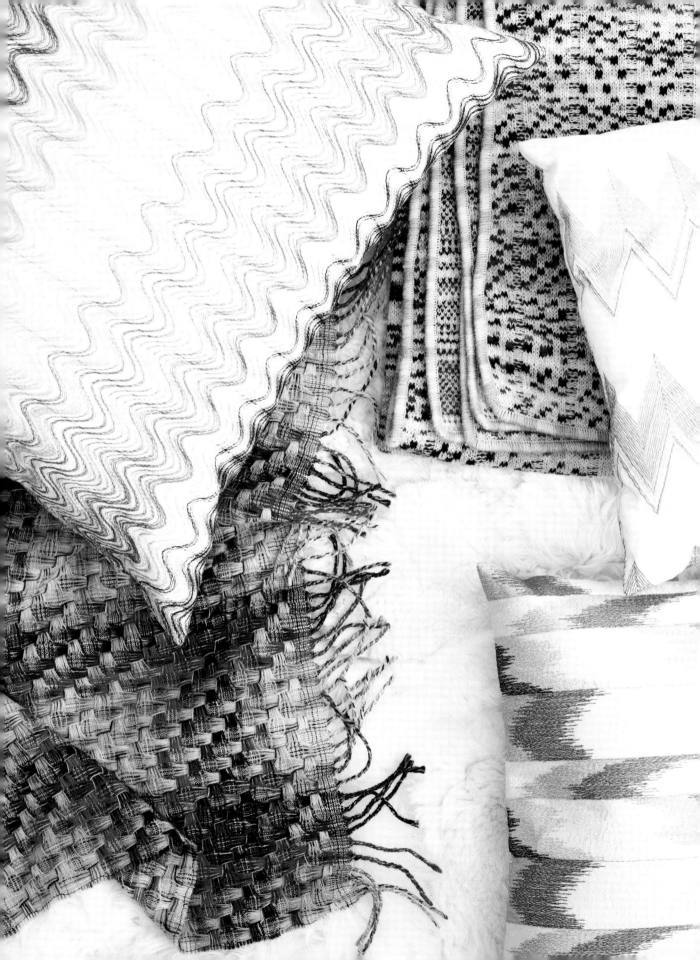

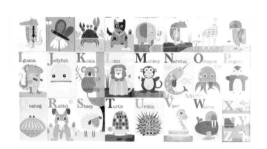

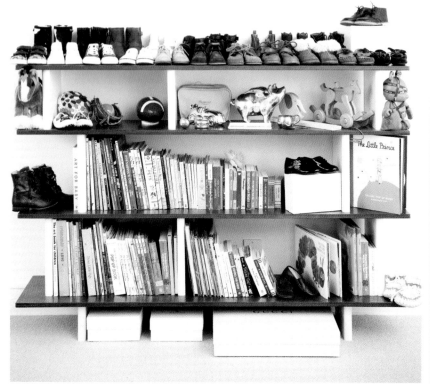

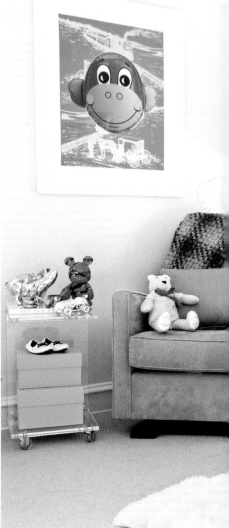

Skyler's nursery

A Chic Nursery

I probably had the most fun when I designed my son's room. All I knew when I first started conceptualizing it was that I wanted Skyler's space to feel dreamy and oasislike to kids and adults alike. The conventional color scheme—pink for a girl, blue for a boy—didn't speak to me. No surprise there, right? Instead, I envisioned a neutral palette with functional modern furniture and accents. His sleek Spot On Square crib was reminiscent of a streamlined Minotti chair, sitting atop a huge sheepskin rug. I can't tell you how many hours the whole family has spent cuddling and reading books on that cloud of a rug, surrounded by his menagerie of plush animals. In addition to a taupe glider, we added an oversized white leather couch that faces the crib from across the room. When

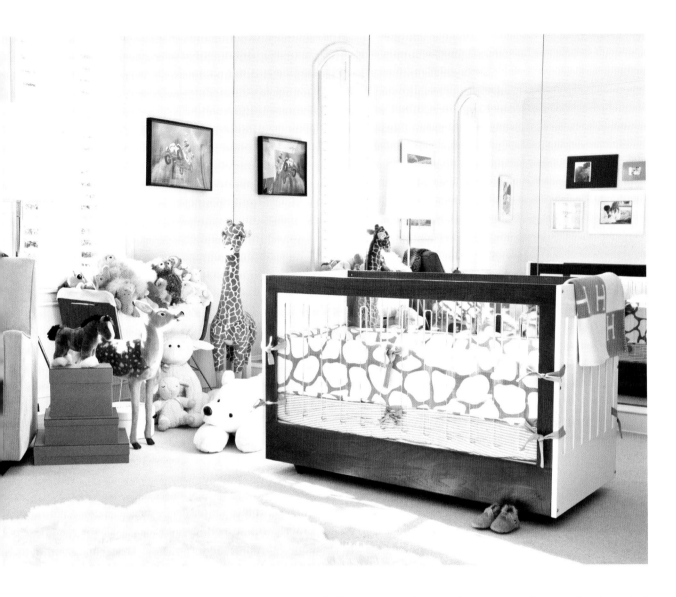

Sky was just a baby and people would come over to see him, I wanted guests to have a place to relax while he played or napped in his crib. Otherwise, everyone lingers around the crib—it can get a little crowded and uncomfortable. It's nice to have a conversation nook in a nursery if you have the space.

What I love most is that his nursery mimics the soothing colors and modern design of the rest of the house. Though that's not to say you won't find stocked bookshelves and rows of his tiny adorable shoes—he also has a stuffed polar bear on display that's almost as big as an armchair! I like to see his silly toys and silver piggy bank when I walk in the door. But his room does feel like a seamless continuation of our décor and as much a part of the house as every other room.

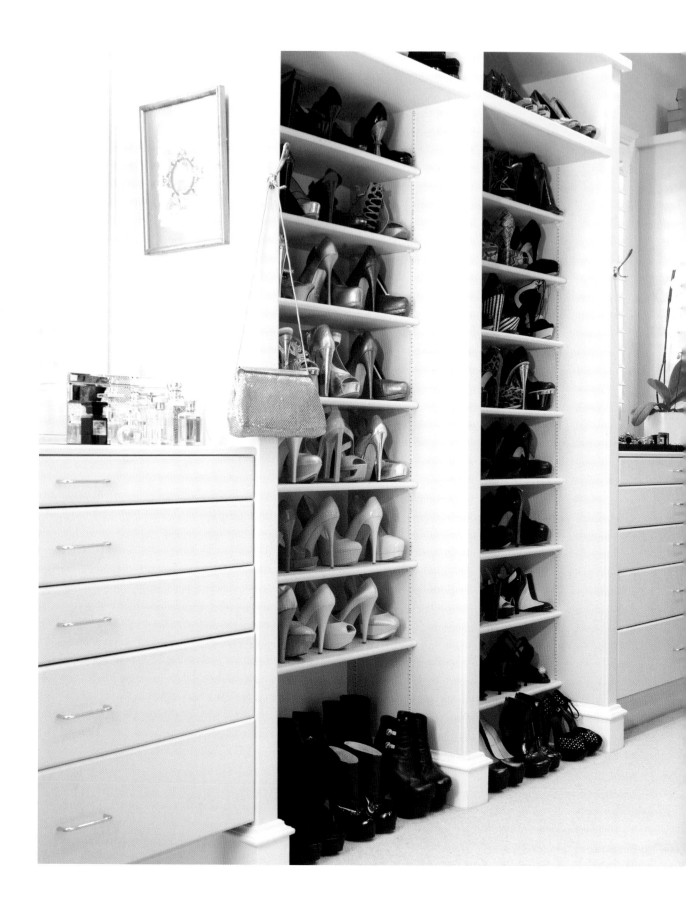

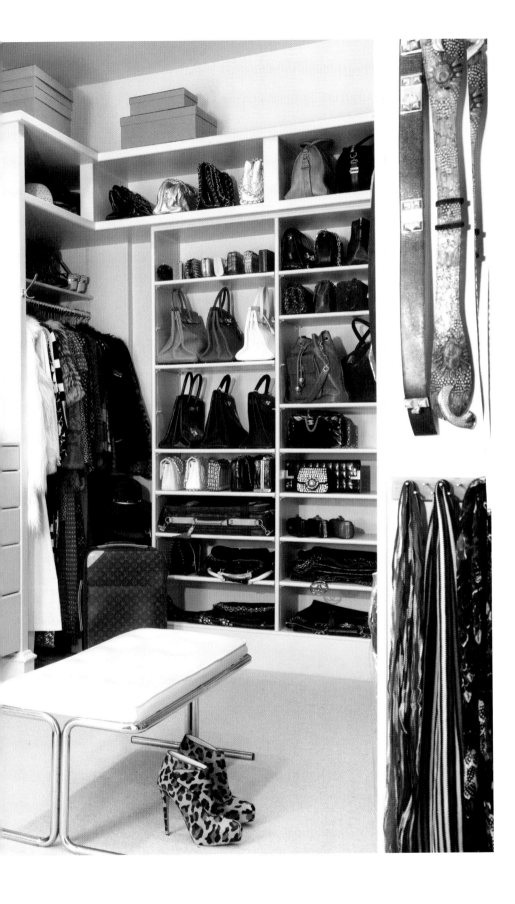

CLOSET CONFIDENTIAL

Nothing makes me more anxious than a disorganized closet, strewn with inside-out clothes, scattered shoes, and puddles of accessories on the floor. Seriously, I hyperventilate. Here's why: As a stylist, one of the first things I learned was the importance of organizing my fashion inventory. Not to mention, ill-handled pieces can easily be damaged. There's nothing more frustrating than trying to untangle a knot of gold chains or discovering that an unworn silk dress needs to be dry-cleaned because it wasn't hung properly.

"NOTHING MAKES ME MORE ANXIOUS THAN A DISORGANIZED CLOSET."

At my headquarters, we have an entire four-thousand-square-foot studio filled with borrowed clothes, shoes, and accessories for red-carpet styling and editorial photo shoots. Every item is categorized according to style, size, designer, and project. We keep files on who wore which piece to what event and when. Jewelry is meticulously logged so that an earring or necklace never gets overlooked. The system must be military in its precision—otherwise we wouldn't be able to operate efficiently.

"THE FIRST THING YOU WOULD SEE IF YOU STEP INTO THE CLOSET OFF MY MASTER BATHROOM IS MY COLLECTION OF CHANEL JACKETS."

Many of the same rules apply to my own closet at home. I'll get into the details of how my closet is arranged in a moment, but I'm not suggesting you must act like a drill sergeant, too. I do know a well-organized wardrobe will make you a more stylish woman, though. If your belts are all raveled into a ball in a bin, it's unlikely you will be able to take the time to pick the best one in the morning. (Instead, hang them from hooks.) Same goes for shoes that can't easily be eyeballed or sweaters that are crammed haphazardly in a stacking cube. Being able to see everything at once makes you more discerning—and who doesn't love options?

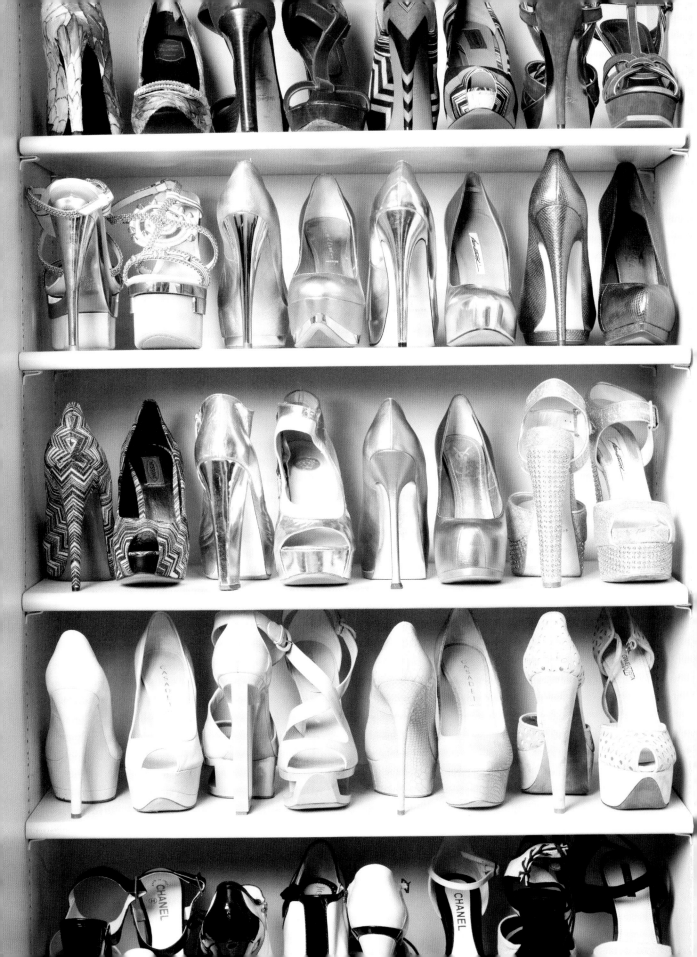

The first thing you would see if you step into the closet off my master bathroom is my collection of Chanel jackets. I like them to be front and center, and I suggest you do the same with your most prized pieces. It's a good rule to spot your favorites right away. New purses that I want to admire are also displayed prominently, outside their dust bags. (I call them "sleeping bags," because I like to think that my purses are cozy and happily resting when they're not with me.) Each pair of shoes sits on a rack with one heel and one toe facing forward so I can assess a shoe's whole look when I'm getting dressed.

Accessories like jewelry and sunglasses have their own shallow slide-out drawers in my closet. My system is built into the closet in matching dressers, but you can invest in valet boxes or clear plastic units with drawers. In my first book, *Style A to Zoe*, I talked about my mom's method of organizing her jewelry in hardware store compartment boxes meant for sorting screws and nails and bolts; I still stand by that practical system.

In addition to my everyday closet, I have racks of clothes that make up my archival collection: vintage pieces with heritage like a Pucci gold lamé gown or a Courrèges peacoat. Some of these clothes are extremely precious and date back more than fifty years. As you can imagine, I handle them with great care and store them accordingly. Sequined pieces are protected with padding on the shoulders so they don't snag other knits and antiquated silks are rolled in acid-free paper.

My overall rules for closet organization are pretty simple and straightforward:

HANG: Choose a uniform hanger style so that all your clothes display at the same level. Wooden ones gobble up inches of space; I prefer a thin version covered in black velvet that prevents slippage. Also, be sure to remove any plastic dry cleaner bags, which trap clothes in the chemicals used in the process. For pants with a center pleat, fold on the crease and clip to hang from the waist.

COORDINATE: Arranging everything—from shoes to dresses to blouses to belts—by color has always worked for me. I find it the easiest way to locate a piece and quickly decide if it suits my palette of the day. Prints and items with sequins, diamantés, or other special embellishments get categorized separately. You might prefer to categorize your pieces according to style, such as skirts or jackets, or to group work and casual wear separately. There are no absolutes when it comes to coordinating your looks, as long as you devote yourself to a system.

FOLD: Certain basics like T-shirts, sweaters, and even jeans are easier to find if you fold and stack them in open-faced cubes rather than pile them in dresser drawers. Just be sure that the stacks you create are not so high they'll topple—I think a maximum of twelve inches is a manageable measure.

STORE: I categorize my intimates and lingerie according to style and then by color and in a drawer, separated with dividers especially made for them. (Fabric-lined organizers are best for delicates.) An open bra clasp can snag on lace, so be sure always to secure them.

PROTECT: I prefer lacquered shelves, but wooden ones should always be covered in paper to avoid splinters and snags. My closet has a few windows, so I'm overly conscious of what's in the path of sunlight. No hats, bags, shoes, or other leather pieces are ever left out to fade. Instead, a pair of white orchids atop my two dressers soaks up the sun.

CHERISH: I know not everyone has a walk-in closet. A few of my apartments in New York had closets with barely enough room for my clothes, let alone me! But if you have the space for a small chair or even an ottoman or bench, I suggest that you create a little perch. It will make you feel all the more glamourous as you decide which shoe or jacket looks major.

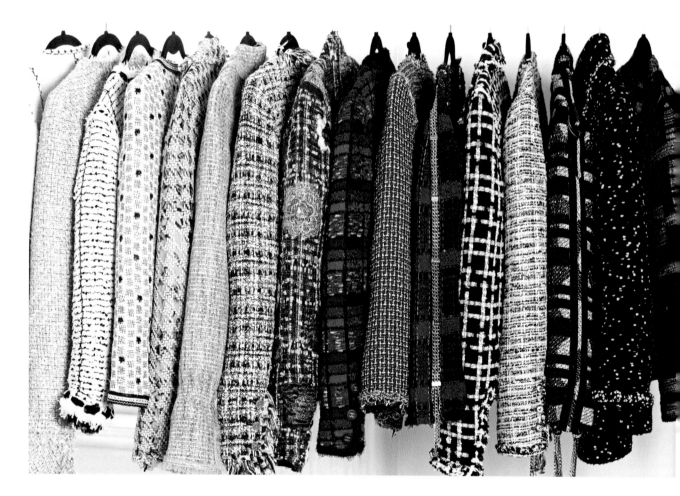

Left: A selection of Chanel jackets from my collection. Right: A selection of sequin pieces from my wardrobe.

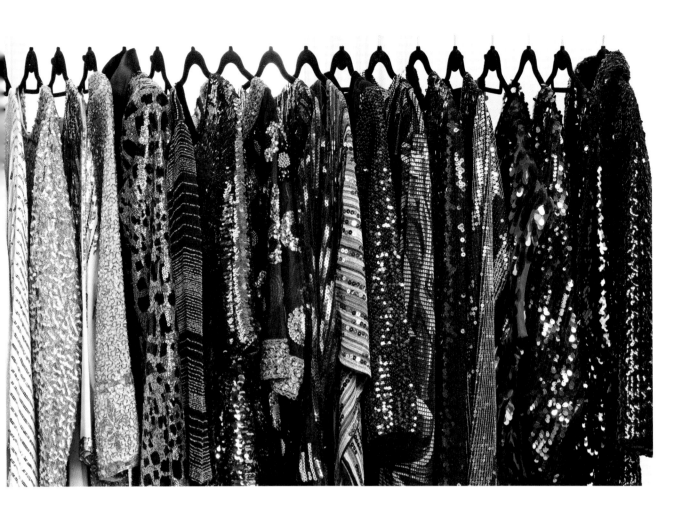

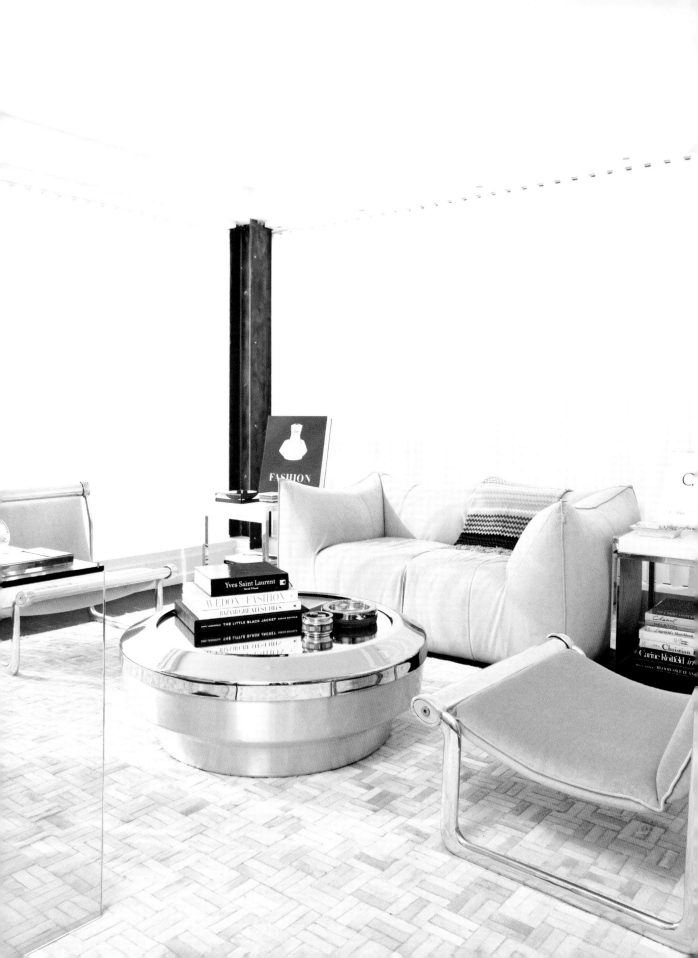

WORKED UP

For years, I worked from my kitchen table wherever I lived. Picture creative colleagues and fashion assistants all sitting in a rectangle, pecking at laptops and taking calls. It was fun, but it's a wonder we ever got anything done at all! A couple of years ago, with my business expanding to include media properties and other ventures, we relocated Rachel Zoe, Inc., to a proper corporate space: a giant, airy loft in an amazing fashion area in West Hollywood on a charming street with chic boutiques and cafés. Suddenly, I had a new all-important challenge: How do I decorate my very first office?

Right away, I knew it had to be a calm, soothing environment. Our days get insane, so I wanted the space to deflect that. My employees would all work at sleek table desks with modern floor lamps and white lacquered credenzas on hand for storage. My own office, situated in a far corner with three walls of glass, needed to be a chic refuge where I could sit and conceptualize a day dress, review my newest collection, or just recharge creatively with a cup of tea. To whittle down my options, I looked to the decades that inspire me as a fashion designer for ideas.

For my own seating, I chose a Knoll wire chair designed by Warren Platner in the 1960s for its comfort and sculptural grace. It also contrasts nicely with my smoked glass table desk, which I try not to clutter. On it, I keep a stack of inspirational art and fashion books alongside a potted cactus and a white orchid. Visitors who pop in can choose between sitting in a Milo Baughman caramel suede and chrome chair from the 1970s or lounging on an off-white Mario Bellini Bambole sofa with peaks like meringue. Thanks to all the natural sunlight and glass walls, I rarely turn on the overhead lights unless I am working late.

The accents here all reflect my taste and infuse my workspace with personality. A white sheepskin rug adds texture and tactile softness, while a throw in black and fuchsia makes for a cheerful pop of color. Adding a small area rug or brightly hued blanket can really help to individualize your area, no matter how large or small the space. A scattering of vintage Gucci ashtrays from the seventies act as little points of interest on my side tables. I do not smoke, but the design of these logo enamel pieces reminds me of that glamourous decade.

Choosing art was a matter of framing inspiration. I knew that I wanted to be able to look up and see some of my style icons. It ultimately came down to black-and-white portraits of Twiggy and Marianne Faithfull, separated by a shot of Halston and Yves Saint Laurent. The collection reminds me to push myself as a fashion designer, and to trust my instincts, too. When you decide on art for your own office or workspace, include images that speak to your creativity. I think a snapshot or two of your family or pet is appropriate, but an entire wall of dog or baby pictures screams that your mind is elsewhere. If you work in a creative field, hang a few portraits of your career idols or of pieces that wow you. As an employer, I like to get a sense of the aspirations and inspirations of my team. Your boss definitely notices those little things.

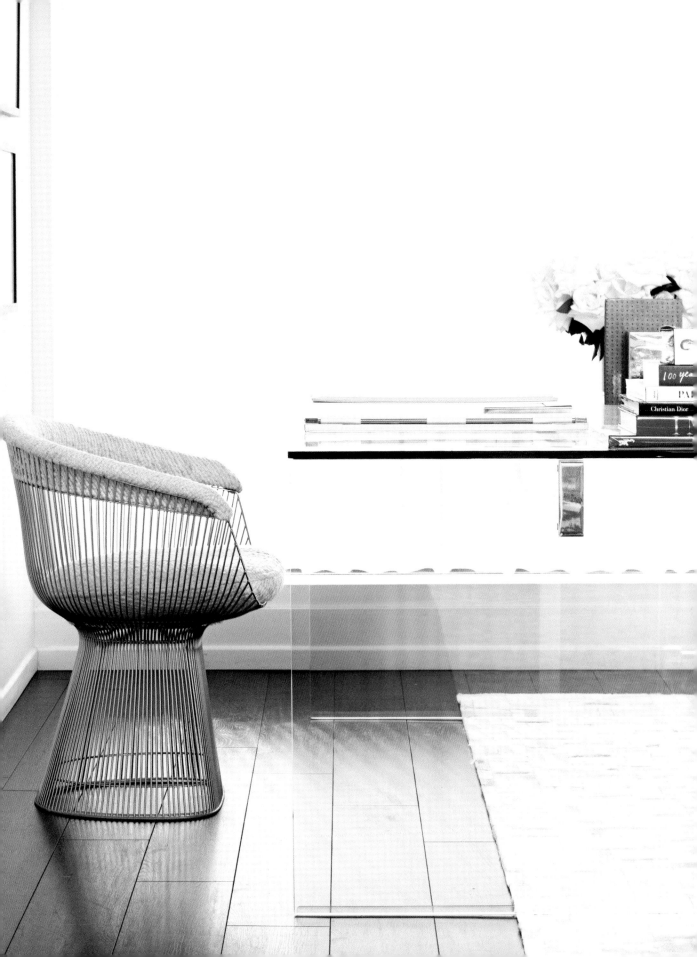

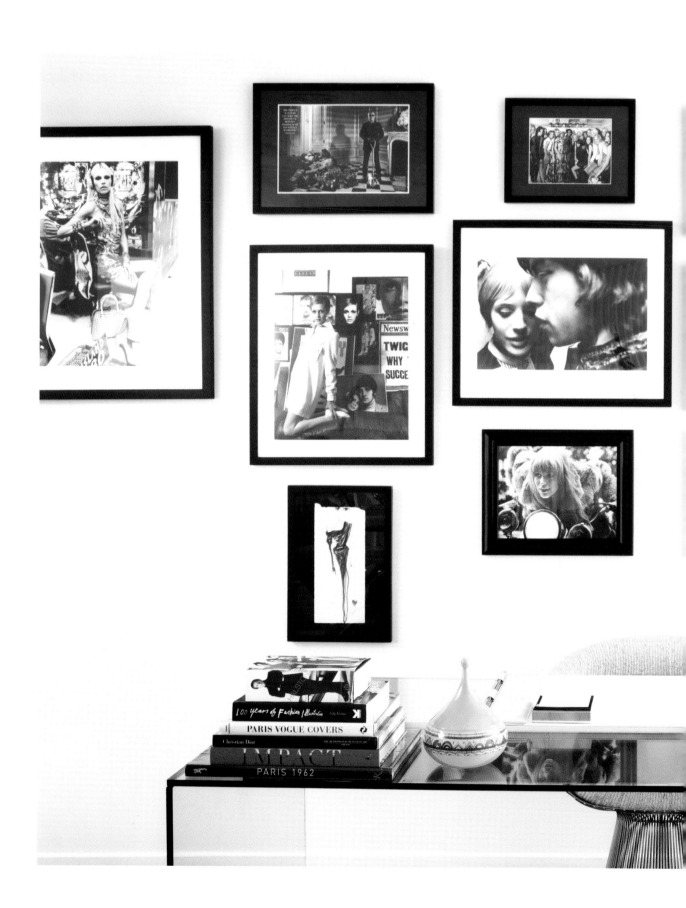

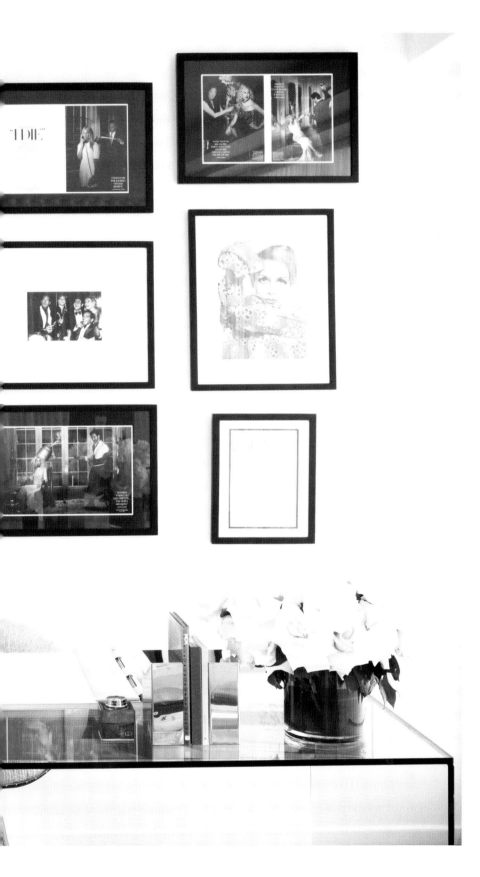

MARTYN LAWRENCE BULLARD
ON HOW TO BUILD A ROOM

With a roster of clients like Cher and Elton John, I have certainly created dramatic and glamourous spaces as an interior decorator. Rachel asked me to share my tips for making a room come together. When I design, I always like to start with the statement piece. In the living room, it's the main sofa, which must be comfortable, inviting, and strong of shape and presence. In a bedroom, it's the bed; in the dining room, it's the table; and so on. Next, I look to the flooring. If possible, I like floorboards dressed with a rug, which adds texture and color. Your floor covering is a great place to pull all the colors in the room together. A fantastic area rug can be put on top of a carpet to add a splash of bold color or a point of interest, too.

Then, start collecting furnishings and don't be afraid to be eclectic. Midcentury modern tables with eighteenth-century chairs on a Pottery Barn sisal rug can be the chicest of combinations. Color, shape, scale, and form are the elements to consider when mixing styles. Color in particular is vital to an interior. It immediately embeds your personal stamp on a space. If your room is dark by nature or has low ceilings, pick a bright color to bring in the sunshine. Consider a brilliant white gloss, Mediterranean turquoise, sunflower yellow, or crisp celadon green. If your room is bright, intense colors will diffuse with the daylight and become inviting at night. Crimson, emerald, cobalt blue, and other jewel tones are great possibilities.

Window dressings add glamour, comfort, and style to a room. Even the most modern abode looks better with some form of window covering, be it glass beads or a sheet of polished steel. Just be sure that they fit in with the character of the space. And lighting is everything. It changes the mood and atmosphere of a room instantly. A statement chandelier or table lamp is truly the jewelry of the space. A dimmer switch, by the way, is an interior designer's best friend!

Personal style is the only real ingredient in a room that matters. Adding personal mementos—like framed photos or trinkets picked up in an exotic market on vacation—is an amazing way to give your room a stylish and inviting vibe. ■

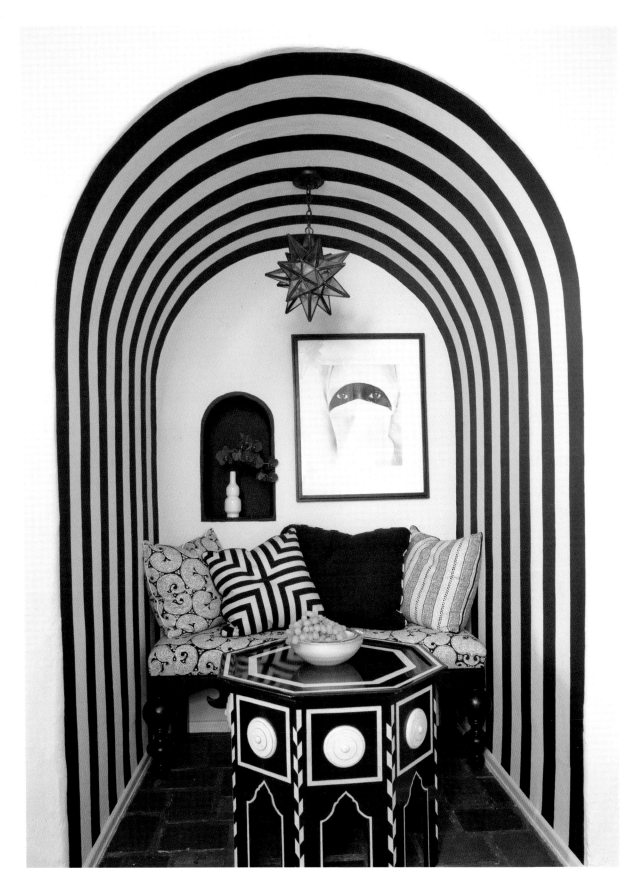

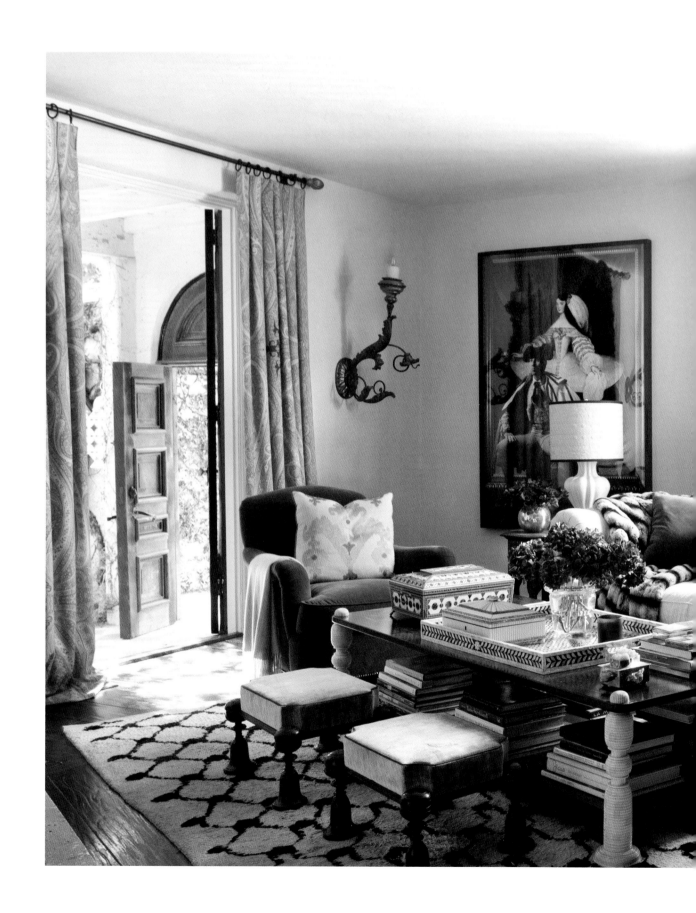

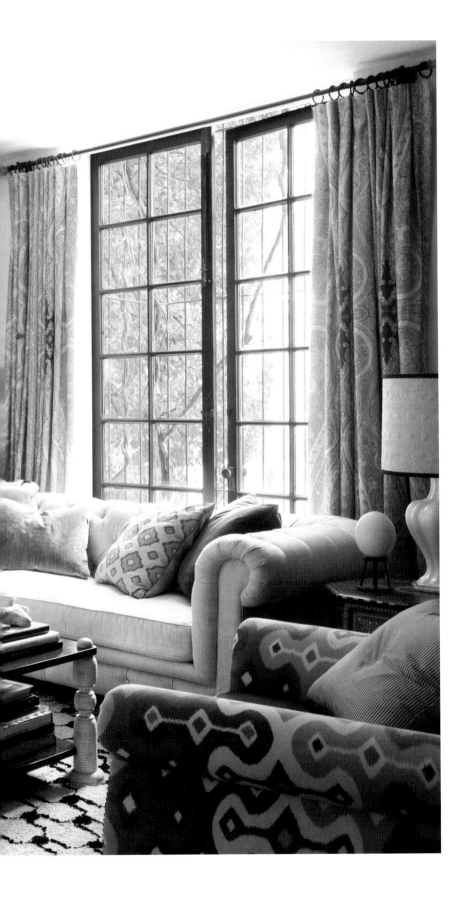

THE GOOD LIFE

Time flies. I know that sounds cliché, but it sometimes feels like just yesterday that I was starting out as a stylist and calling in a couture gown for the first time (twenty years ago!), or that Rodger and I were talking until dawn on our very first date (I was nineteen then, by the way). Of course, those two moments became amazing life milestones—discovering my passion and meeting my best friend—so they will always resonate with me. And thankfully, I met a man who is as crazy about celebrating life as I am. We also savor the more low-key happenings, too. Rituals and traditions have always been a big deal for us.

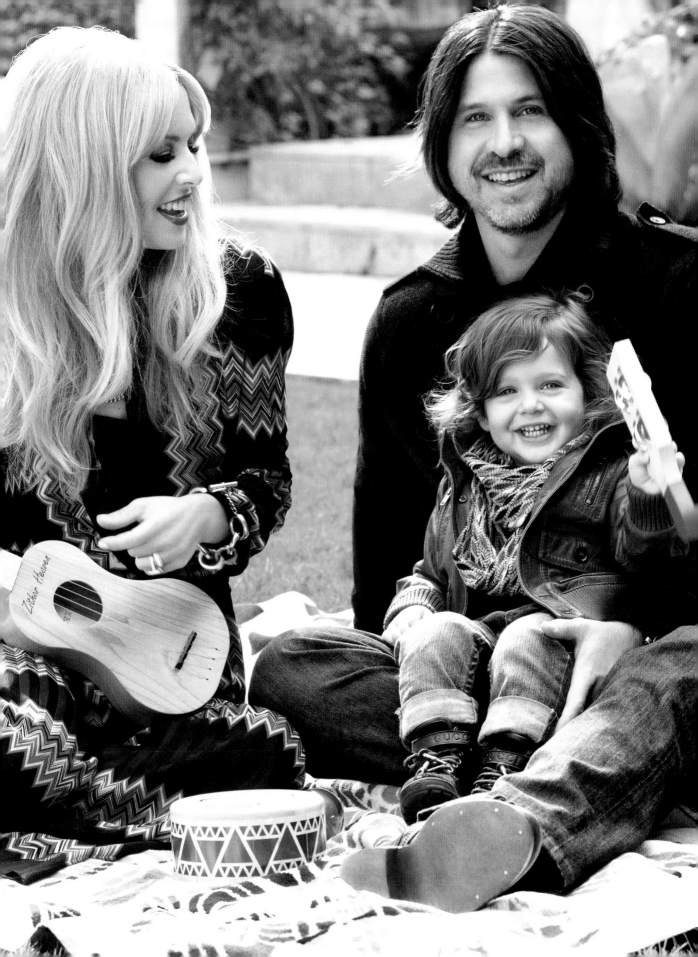

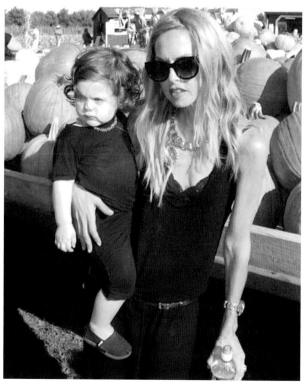
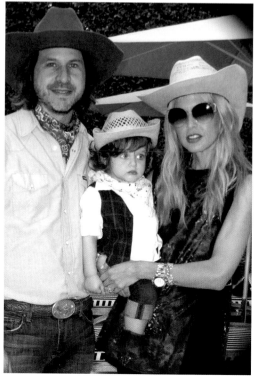
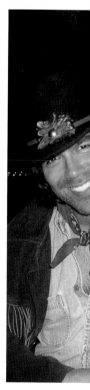

Left: With Skyler at the farmer's market, 2012. Center: With Rodger and Skyler on Halloween, 2012. Right: With Brian Atwood, 2010.

These days, it's harder for people to commit to quality time, because we are all so incredibly busy. You might be juggling the demands of a job with the needs of your family. Or you may be spending every free hour updating a style blog—and I just might be following it, too. Technology has forced us all to become master multitaskers. We work, we sleep, we worry about what we didn't manage to do! Who isn't always playing catch-up? Trust me, I know what it's like to overschedule yourself.

"SOMETIMES, THOUGH, YOU HAVE TO PUT ASIDE THE TO-DO LIST AND RAISE A GLASS TO ALL THE GOOD THINGS IN LIFE."

Sometimes, though, you have to put aside the to-do list and raise a glass to all the good things in life. I'm not talking just about major holidays or anniversaries. Growing up, my family sat down for dinner together almost every night. At the time, it was hard for me to understand why we needed to spend an hour at the dining room table when I could have been on the phone with my friends or flipping through *Vogue*. Now, as an adult, I understand why my mom and dad insisted on this time and I have carried it on to my own family.

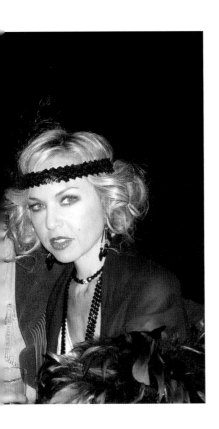

It's the simplest rituals that you come to value the most in life. Every Sunday, for instance, Rodger, Skyler, and I all go to our local farmer's market in Beverly Hills and spend an hour or so browsing the stands and picking up fresh fruit and vegetables for the week. Sky nibbles on ripe berries while I shop for orchids and organic greens like mesclun and arugula. Not only has this become a regular family outing, but also one of the highlights of my week.

"IT'S THE SIMPLEST RITUALS THAT YOU COME TO VALUE THE MOST IN LIFE."

No doubt, every year will bring new traditions. My feelings toward certain occasions have changed, too. I never used to care about Halloween, but once you have a child, it becomes very important, as you can imagine. When Sky was one and a half, we all dressed up as cowboys and visited a pumpkin patch. We had the best time! And I imagine we'll keep it up until he outgrows it. But of course, I reserve my chic flapper costume for the nighttime parties.

We also recently started hosting a major family Thanksgiving feast at our house. And the same goes for Passover—I'm talking up to twenty people. Full disclosure: I may not cook all day (you'll learn more about how I entertain in Chapter 7), but I've found my own way to honor these holidays. When I look around the table and see my family and friends, I feel lucky to have such amazing people in my life. In the end, it's all about enjoying as much as we possibly can.

Obviously, I can't stop time, but I *can* make every moment as memorable as possible. The past few years have brought more responsibilities for me as a mom and within my career. And the busier I get, the more I realize how important it is to appreciate life and make the most of it. I hope you will be inspired by this peek into how I make merry on some of my favorite occasions.

LOVE ALWAYS

As I said earlier, I can still recall every minute of my first date with Rodger—even though it lasted almost eight hours! The cutest part? When he dropped me off after we talked most of the night, he asked, "Do you want to see me tomorrow?" (I said yes!) We haven't been apart many days since that night on August 29, 1991.

Over the years, so much has changed. We moved across the country, built a company together, and started a family. I like to say that Rodger and I are both codependent and independent. We completely live for each other and need each other, but we can also exist separately. In my mind, that independence is the most important aspect of a successful relationship or marriage. In order to thrive independently, you need to have a solid and unshakable trust—an assurance that allows you always to be yourself. Rodger has seen a vulnerable side of me that I rarely show to anyone and sometimes I need to be strong for him, too. In my experience, you must take turns being strong and supportive for each other.

As you could probably guess, romantic holidays are a big deal for us. Every year, we celebrate both the night of our first date and our wedding anniversary. In August, we're usually away on vacation and enjoy a simple dinner out together. But our wedding anniversary is a little more of a tradition: Because we got married on February 15, we usually skip going out on Valentine's Day and opt for a night of pizza and movies with our single friends. Little did I know when I married Rodger that our anniversary would fall right in the middle of Fashion Week and so close to Oscar season—not exactly a low-key time for me. For the past decade or so, we've had a New York tradition of going to see Marc Jacobs's runway show and then dashing over to Babbo—Mario Batali's fantastic flagship restaurant—for a romantic late-night supper.

A couple of years ago, Rodger wowed me with a romantic getaway to the Beverly Hills Hotel for our twenty-first anniversary, post–Fashion Week. Okay, so the hotel is only a few blocks from our house, but it's a rare night that we aren't with Skyler. I walked into a gorgeous suite to find Champagne, chocolates, and rose petals scattered everywhere. What an amazing night. I even quoted Julia Roberts from *Pretty Woman* and said to my husband, "If I forget to tell you later, I had a wonderful time tonight."

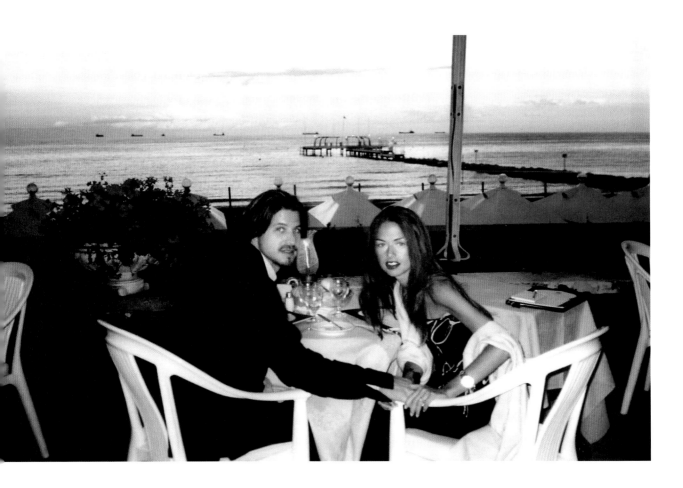

*With Rodger in
Santorini, 1991*

After all these years and celebrations, you might think that Rodger and I
have run out of ideas for gifts. No way. I'm fanatical about buying presents
for everyone in my life, so each year I listen for clues on what my husband
might want. (Keep in mind that the stakes are high, as this is a man who
left a trail of rose petals that led to a giant orange Hermès box on my thir-
tieth birthday—it was my first Birkin.)

Over the course of our relationship, I have surprised Rodger with simple
silver jewelry, vintage watches, golf bags, and engraved ID bracelets. One
of my most recent gifts to him was a chic Linus roadster bicycle, mod-
eled after a 1950s French design. He nearly cried when I wheeled it out,
because he had casually mentioned that he wanted a bike, but didn't think
that it registered with me. One year I gave Rodger a chic picture frame with
a photo of him holding Skyler. He later gave me the same style of frame
with a picture of Sky and me. In a way, we were acknowledging that our
son was the ultimate gift that we gave to each other. Just thinking about
those frames reminds me that exchanging gifts is really more about being
thoughtful than buying something extravagant.

THE BIG DAY

Everyone is entitled to their own red-carpet moments, and your wedding is definitely the most important. It's your day to be the center of attention and shine. Initially, I thought I wanted to marry Rodger somewhere exotic with family and just a few friends. I envisioned a beach or cliff side in the South of France or Positano. But my father was so excited for us and wanted to celebrate with an unforgettable event. In the end, we decided to throw a black-tie party at the Rainbow Room in Manhattan in 1998. My bridesmaids wore black velvet gowns with gloves and my wedding dress was this gorgeous Isaac Mizrahi gown with a fitted bodice and tulle skirt. I had seen the gown in red on the cover of *Vogue* and I called Isaac to beg him to make it for me in white. (I was on hold for thirty minutes pacing back and forth while I waited for his decision. It felt like hours!)

"IF I CAN SHARE ANY ADVICE, IT'S SIMPLY TO MAKE SURE YOU HOLD HANDS WITH YOUR PARTNER AS MUCH AS YOU CAN AT YOUR WEDDING."

In hindsight, I'm glad our wedding was a glamourous affair. I felt like a princess during every moment of it. Everywhere I turned, our dearest friends and family were dancing and toasting our happiness. It was truly the most magical night of my life. If I can share any advice, it's simply to make sure you hold hands with your partner as much as you can at your wedding. It's easy to get separated when you're making the rounds and greeting your guests. Everyone wants to talk to you! Rodger and I even stepped away right after the ceremony to enjoy a private moment and look out at the people who were there with us. I can't even remember what we said to each other—only that neither of us could stop smiling.

BRIDAL CHIC

Obviously, I couldn't mention weddings without discussing *the dress*. When you flip through your photo album thirty years from now, you should still love it as much as you did on your special day. I have styled all different types of brides, from a friend who married in a slip dress in a Kansas cornfield to an actress who literally toppled over trying on a giant tulle ball gown. Of course, the silhouette and style you choose should suit your personality and the ambience of the wedding itself—but I always suggest going more classic than contemporary.

How to find the perfect gown? Before anything else, go through tons of magazines and books to look at as many gowns as you can. I also advise you to begin pulling clips from magazines about six months before you even start shopping. A bridal salon can be incredibly overwhelming if you don't have a general sense of what you want to wear. *But,* at the same time, be open to anything. Yes, in essence, you are preparing to ultimately change your mind. It sounds crazy, but I have found that most women wear the opposite of what they assumed would feel right on them.

"WHEN IT COMES TO ACCESSORIES, I HAVE THREE WORDS FOR YOU: WEAR A VEIL."

When it comes to accessories, I have three words for you: Wear a veil. My philosophy is that you have one day in your life to do it, so take advantage of that opportunity. It's romantic and timeless and makes the walk down the aisle a true Cinderella moment. If you're worried about comfort, you can always take it off right after the ceremony. Wear a pair of shoes that are comfortable, too, so that you can dance all night. Stash wedges or lower heels under the table if you think you'll need to make a quick switch. As for jewelry, choose classic styles over dramatic pieces. It's tempting to wear an over-the-top necklace or chandelier earrings, but you don't want your gems to compete with your wedding dress. Even a simple slip dress shouldn't be upstaged by big jewelry. I typically recommend that brides select accessories close to their everyday style. If you always wear gold hoops, try on a pair with pavé diamonds. I opted for classic diamond solitaire studs.

With bridal beauty, again, be true to your style. If you don't typically wear a lot of makeup, do a natural, glamourous look for your wedding—just amp it up a little bit. Remember: You want to feel comfortable and look like yourself.

You may be seduced by trends, but on this occasion, I always recommend that you veer more toward traditional. Believe me, I have seen brides make outlandish decisions just because they saw it on a runway or in a bridal magazine. You just might regret the purple leather opera gloves or that mini top hat. If you feel the need to distinguish yourself with a unique accent, opt for a subtle highlight like a colored sash or shoes. When it's right, you'll know it.

Next spread: Our wedding day, February 15, 1998

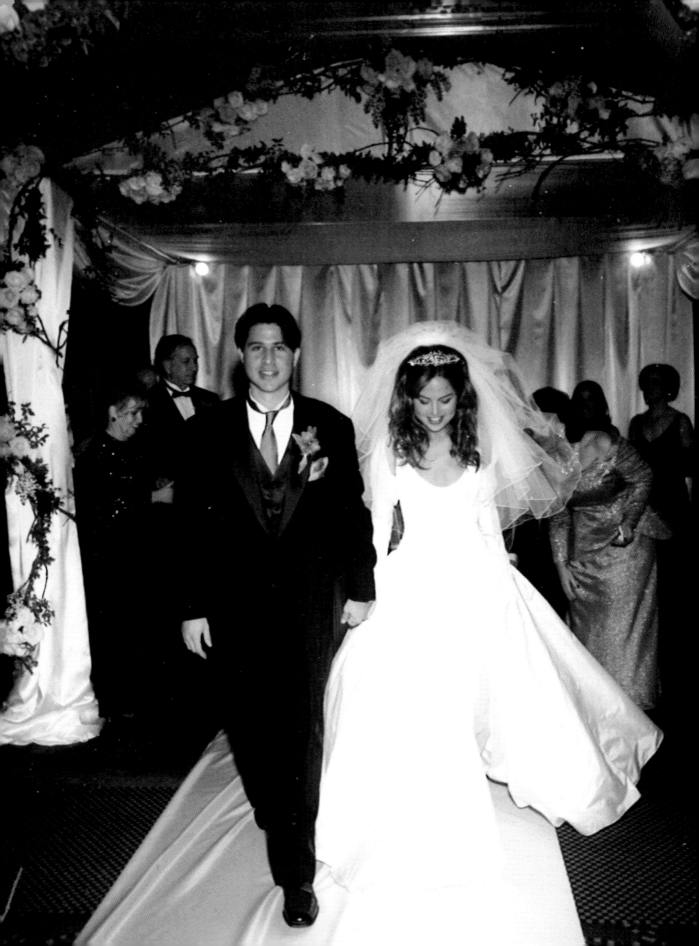

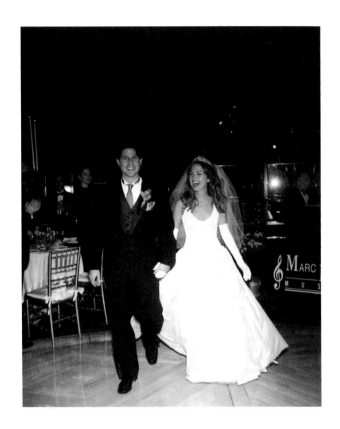

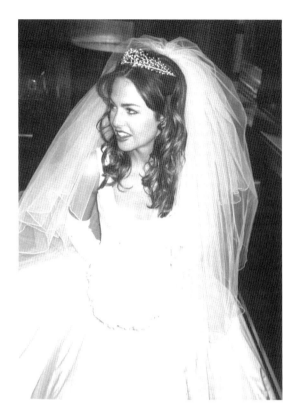

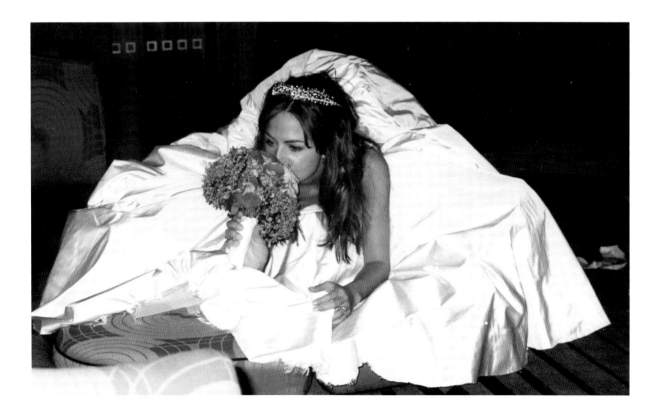

VIP DAYS

Every year, I insist that I am doing something "small" for my birthday—no matter my age. "I don't want anything over the top," I will say to Rodger. But then, about a week before the big day, I suddenly realize that I miss my friends and want to throw a huge, amazing party just to see them all. At this point, Rodger is so used to my indecisiveness that he scouts out a space and reserves it for when I decide I do want to have a party. If you're on the fence about whether or not to make something into an occasion, I say go for it. You never want to regret a missed opportunity to make a lasting memory—for yourself and for the people you love.

"IF YOU'RE ON THE FENCE ABOUT WHETHER OR NOT TO MAKE SOMETHING INTO AN OCCASION, I SAY GO FOR IT. YOU NEVER WANT TO REGRET A MISSED OPPORTUNITY TO MAKE A LASTING MEMORY—FOR YOURSELF AND FOR THE PEOPLE YOU LOVE."

For my fortieth birthday—a big deal, I know—we took over a bungalow at the Chateau Marmont in West Hollywood. This effortlessly chic and legendary hotel has always been a favorite of mine. Rodger and a few friends even put together a slide show of photos that made me cry and then laugh and then cry again. (Why didn't I burn those pictures of me from the eighties when I had the chance?) We all got dressed up and danced until our feet ached. When the moment felt right, I stood up and gave a quick toast to my guests. At any event I host, I try to express my gratitude to my guests by letting them know how much they all mean to me. It's been a tradition of mine for as long as I can remember—I believe I even spoke at my birthday parties when I was a little girl! I don't think you ever need a reason to be thankful for your health and happiness. When it comes to public speaking, my motto is this: Speak from the heart. When Rodger speaks at a party, the whole room freezes, because he's so captivating. His roast to my mom at her sixtieth birthday had people laughing all night and his toast to me on my thirty-fifth birthday received a standing ovation.

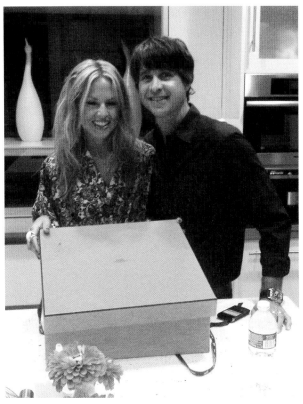

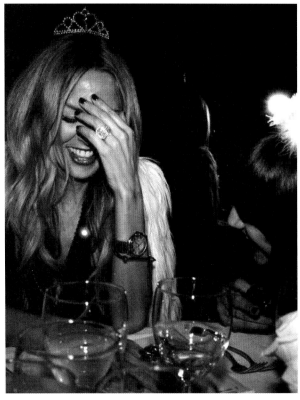

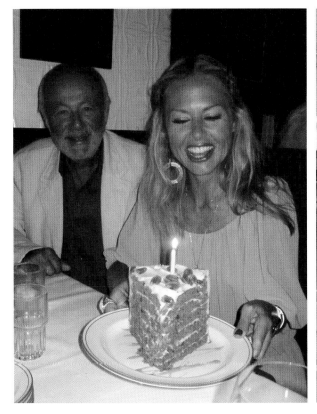

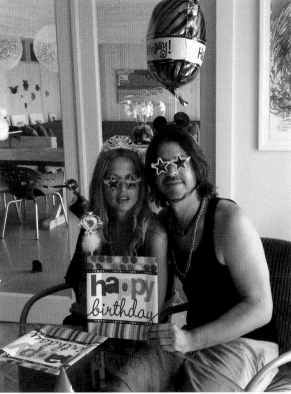

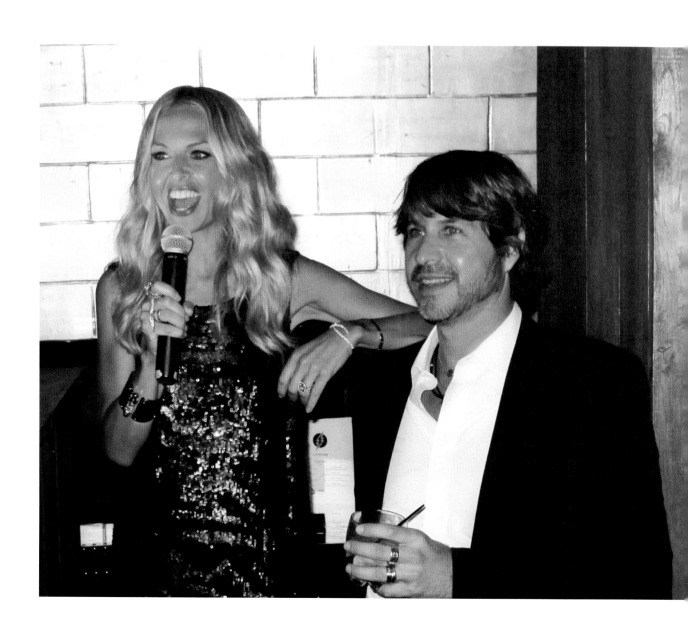

RODGER BERMAN ON GIVING A GREAT TOAST

Rachel's birthday party every year is a chance to publicly acknowledge what she means to me and tell her how proud I am of her evolution. I don't write down what I plan to say, but I do spend a few hours thinking about it beforehand and try to formulate a beginning, middle, and end.

HIT ON A COMMON THEME. The most important thing to remember is that you want the audience to feel included. If you tell a personal story about someone, make sure you tap into a known personality trait or experience that is familiar to everyone.

SURPRISE EVERYONE. Sometimes, I also like to reveal a side of someone's nature that might not be so evident. For instance, one year, I thanked Rachel for making breakfast for me every morning. Not everyone realizes that she's such a caretaker; it was nice to be able to point that out.

HUMOR ALWAYS WORKS. Everyone loves to laugh at a party or wedding. My toasts are usually more heartfelt than humorous, but I am known for making some sly references and gently poking fun at someone or a situation.

READ YOUR AUDIENCE. Rachel keeps her speeches to a minute or two, but I tend to go on longer. I don't think you want to talk for more than five minutes, though. It's always smart to look out at the guests and read their faces and body language. If people are fidgeting or not making eye contact with you, wrap it up. ■

Top and bottom, left:
Skyler with his family on
his first birthday. Bottom
right: With Rodger and
Skyler at our Memorial
Day barbecue.

KID STUFF

Why is it that children's birthday parties have become a competitive sport? I like to think it's because parents want their kids to have *the* best day. My philosophy is this: Children are happy with simple snacks, some upbeat music, and lots of smiling faces. Ponies and petting zoos are fun, but certainly not essential. When Skyler turned one, we planned a little party in the backyard that soon ballooned to a hundred guests. What was that I said about going big? But when it rained that morning, we moved it indoors at a nearby restaurant and brought in a face painter and a music teacher who got everyone jumping around and dancing. Trust me, my son is an excellent dancer! If you want to go for it, that's fine, but no one should feel pressured to spend a small fortune to hire a circus for a group of toddlers. At the end of the day, a balloon and cake make any kid happy.

THE ANNUAL BBQ

Remember how much you loved sleepovers and pool parties as a kid simply for the joy of spending time with your friends? It didn't matter that you saw them every day at school. As adults, we sometimes outgrow that urge to invite people over just because we love them, but you never need a reason to gather your friends and family.

Every year, about three weeks before Memorial Day, Rodger and I start to get e-mails asking, "What time is the barbecue?" and phone messages like, "Can't wait! What can we bring?" It's a running joke—or rather, known fact—among our friends that we will host a BBQ on the inaugural summer holiday every year. We've been throwing this bash for about five years now, and I have a feeling it will be a lifelong Berman family tradition.

Initially, this barbecue was a small, intimate gathering of eight or ten close friends. But every year, it never fails that the guest list expands, making our small barbecue into an all-day soiree for fifty! (Are you seeing a theme here?) Truthfully, it's better this way—we get to spend the afternoon with so many people we adore. I always say if you're going to do the prep work for a party, you may as well make it a major one! We get to see everyone we care about all at once, and include them as part of what has become one of our favorite rituals, too.

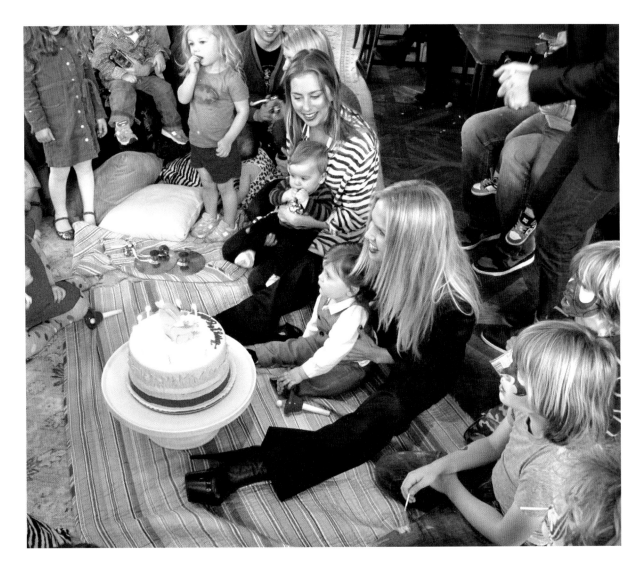

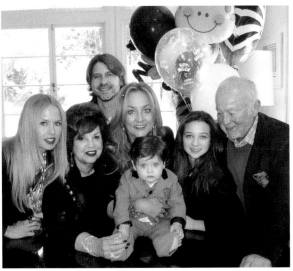

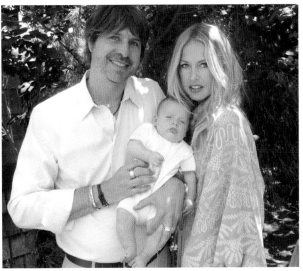

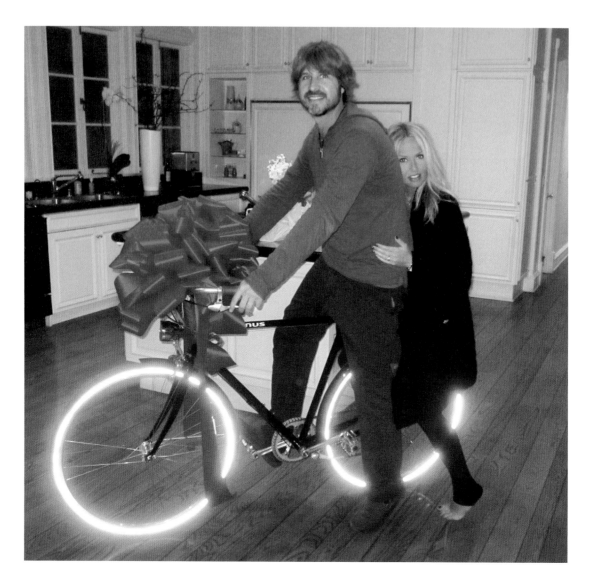

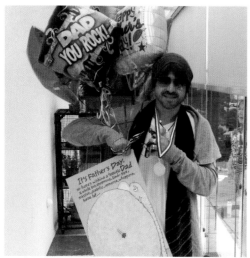

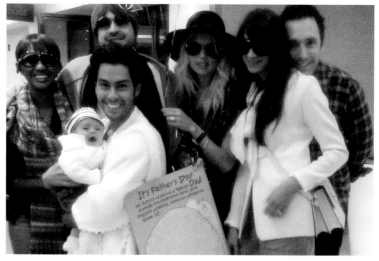

Top: Rodger's first Father's Day gift. Bottom: Rodger's first Father's Day.

FATHER'S DAY

Growing up, Father's Day was always a big deal for me. I had a "Daddy's Little Girl" nightgown that I wore until I outgrew it. Every year, I woke up early to make my father a special omelet and pancakes. Now that my husband is a father, too, I like to thank him for being such an incredible dad to Skyler. That usually means a special brunch and a day at the park. For his first Father's Day, a group of friends joined us for brunch and we made him wear a goofy "Number One Dad" sash and hat. In true Rodger form, he wasn't embarrassed in the least. And Skyler giggled nonstop!

FRIENDSHIPS FOREVER

As important and fun as these big gatherings are, my close girlfriends also mean everything to me. Unfortunately, with our insane schedules, it's difficult for us to find time to get together. And I know that we're not the only women who need to send at least a dozen e-mails to organize a dinner. Since our free time is so limited and we want to make the most of our few hours together, we usually make it a "girls' night in." If it's at my house, I might order a spread of Mexican food and make flavored margaritas. If we decide to bring in pizzas and chopped salads, I'll open a few bottles of Chianti and Pinot Grigio. Some nights, we just lounge around and catch up on what's happening with each other. But I have a few more fun ideas for making the most of your girls' night.

RED WINE, RED NAILS. If you're like me, you can barely find time to get to a nail salon. Hire a few local nail technicians who can do quickie manicures for an hour or two. Catching up with friends while you sip wine and get pampered feels so luxurious and decadent.

PUSH PLAY. My girlfriends and I used to meet every week to watch *Gossip Girl* together at one of our houses. We would order takeout and hit pause a million times to discuss every amazing outfit and steamy scene. (I actually did a cameo in one episode, in which a vat of chocolate ended up on my head and my Pucci dress. Insane!) Now that show has ended, but we try to get together for a regular movie night instead. I love to screen a favorite film like *Almost Famous*. Who doesn't love Kate Hudson's fabulous seventies groupie costumes?

DO GOOD, FEEL GOOD. Every once in a while, we gather to talk about charities or causes that are important to us. We might discuss how to raise awareness or brainstorm on planning an event. A few times, we have even volunteered together as our girls' night activity. One organization in particular, Baby2Baby, is close to my heart, because they supply families in need with baby gear and essentials. I'm also an ambassador to the incredible foundation Save the Children. Why not have a little fun with philanthropy?

"BANANAS" BREAD RECIPE

When I need to get zen, I bake—maybe it's the precision required in measuring and mixing ingredients that soothes me. During the frantic weeks leading up to Fashion Week and award season, I have been known to bake dozens of cookies and brownies for my office. It has become such a tradition that my team starts to drop not-so-subtle hints like "Where is your apron?" No matter what, it's always my chocolate chip banana bread that disappears the fastest.

½ cup softened unsalted butter, plus more for greasing the pan
1 cup sugar
2 eggs
1 cup mashed bananas (about 3 medium overripe)
2 cups all-purpose flour
1 teaspoon baking powder
½ teaspoon baking soda
½ teaspoon salt
1 cup milk chocolate or semisweet chocolate chips (optional)
½ cup walnuts, peanuts, or pecans (optional)

- Heat oven to 350°F. Lightly grease the bottom of a 9 x 5 x 3–inch loaf pan (do not grease sides).

- Beat the ½ cup butter and the sugar in large bowl with electric mixer on medium speed until fluffy (about one minute). Beat in the eggs and bananas until smooth (about one more minute). Add the flour, baking powder, baking soda, and salt, and beat, just until mixed. Stir in the chocolate chips and nuts with a spatula, if using.

- Pour the mixture into the prepared pan. Bake for 1 hour and 10 minutes or until a toothpick comes out clean.

- Allow the bread to cool in the pan for 10 minutes and then remove it to a wire rack. Allow it to cool completely, about 1 hour.

For an even more decadent finish, I sometimes add a crumble topping:

½ cup sugar
⅓ cup all-purpose flour
½ teaspoon cinnamon
¼ cup softened unsalted butter

Mix all the ingredients together until crumbly, then sprinkle over the loaf for the last 30 minutes of baking.

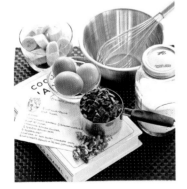

"Bananas" Bread ingredients

CHAPTER 7

LET'S HAVE A PARTY

Someone at a dinner party once asked me to name my top five wish-list dinner guests alive or not. What a great question, right? My mind somersaulted because there are *so many* people I would want to invite!

To me, creating a guest list is a lot like building your wardrobe. You want to include your trusted go-tos and something a bit unexpected while always maintaining a perfect balance. Those are my considerations when I fantasize about my dream dinner party.

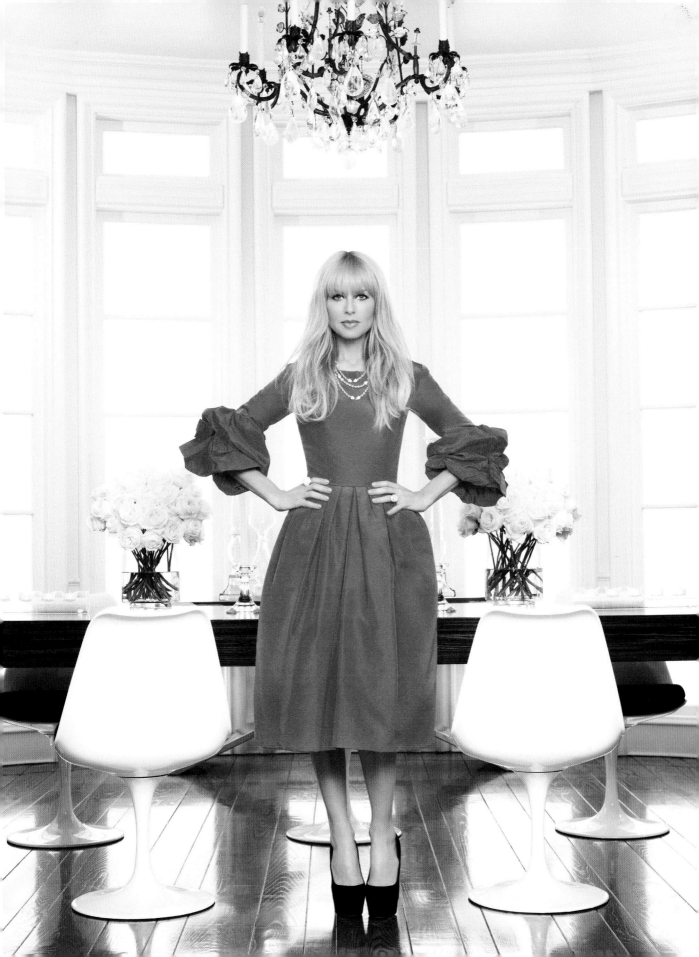

First of all, Brigitte Bardot would *have* to come—she's so private. but I think she would really open up in this intimate setting. Coco Chanel would receive an invite, too. She led an unbelievably fascinating life and I could ask her all sorts of questions about her philosophies on fashion, men, and Paris society. I would absolutely include Jane Birkin, and seat her to my right. She's the most fabulous woman in the world without even trying. I would ask her about the swinging sixties in London—she and Bardot could reminisce about the sexy film *Don Juan* that they made together in 1973. Of course, I would be a fool to pass up a chance to invite a Beatle. Paul McCartney is my pick. He could even sing a few songs during dessert. Then, there's Johnny Depp. I have had a crush on this brilliant actor since I was thirteen and I know he's a perpetually captivating person. He has managed to maintain his personal style and integrity as an actor—an amazing and admirable feat.

This imaginary dinner party would be amazing, but how would I prepare for such fabulous guests? In my last chapter, I shared my favorite rituals and holidays. Now, it's time to talk about *how* to throw together a gathering— and why parties for no particular reason might be my favorite ones of all.

THE ART OF BEING AN EXCELLENT HOSTESS

When it comes to entertaining, I learned a long time ago that trying to accomplish everything invariably leads to a disaster. You know that hostess, the one who's smiling a little too wide and looks like she is about to have a nervous breakdown in the kitchen? Maybe she just burned the risotto and she's trying to keep it together. Or she was so busy that she never had a chance to shower and she's wearing last night's mascara. Unfortunately, guests pick up on that energy and then feel like they're imposing. I should know, because I have been that frazzled hostess once or twice—but not anymore.

The key to being a fantastic entertainer is to look like you are having an amazing time—because you really *are* enjoying yourself, of course. If that means ordering in a spread and just mixing the cocktails and pouring the wine, do that. Your friends don't come to your home to judge you on your ability to whip up foie gras or make the perfect roast chicken. One Thanksgiving, I dashed around the kitchen like a crazed French chef and served a twelve-pound turkey with a slew of side dishes. (Of course, I was

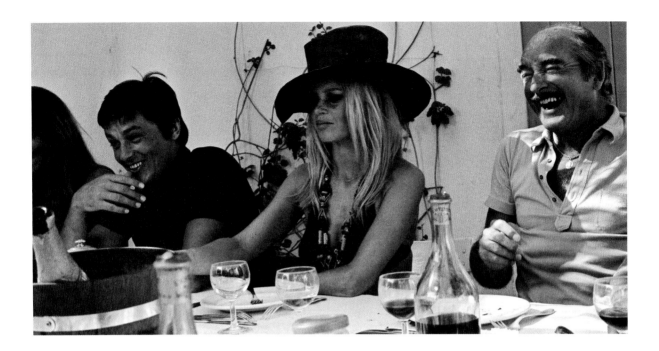

Brigitte Bardot at a dinner party

wearing a turban, but no apron.) It was rewarding, but completely exhausting. Though I hope my guests did, I didn't get to enjoy the occasion as much as I would have liked, because I was so busy.

Lately, my party MO is to oversee a few hors d'oeuvres—including my grandmother's insanely beloved baked salami roll—and to roast almonds in the oven, which makes the whole house smell welcoming and festive. Instead of creating the entire menu, I usually have the main dishes catered so that I can enjoy myself, especially now that I have Sky on my hip and everyone wants to play with him. I also set out what I can early in the day so there's time to shower and to dress up before guests arrive.

Still, even the most meticulous groundwork doesn't guarantee everything will go as planned. I have burned that baked salami a few times—but a little char actually makes it taste better, believe it or not. Even if I do make a mistake (and we all do), I don't let it destroy my night. I just laugh and admit to my guests that I dried out the chicken and that we need to order out. I'm the first to ask "Okay, who wants Thai?" You have to see the humor in any situation—whether it's a sudden downpour at your barbecue or a salty soufflé. Everyone else will follow your lead and laugh, too.

As a hostess, my entertaining checklist is fairly simple and straightforward. I try not to focus on the little details—which no one else notices anyway—and direct my energy to the elements that matter most to me.

KEEP THE LIGHTING DIM AND FLATTERING. Unless it's natural sunlight, an overly bright setting is not only unkind to anyone over the age of twenty-five, but it also makes you feel like you're dining in a department store. Candlelight—from dainty flickering votives to magnificent pillars—always delivers a warm glow that makes everyone look like they just returned from a weekend in Saint-Tropez. For fixtures in the dining room, look for incandescent bulbs that emit a soft amber light instead of harsh white with blue undertones. I'm a huge fan of dimmers, which are fantastic for adjusting mood lighting. If you don't have dimmers, opt for lamplight instead of overhead, and strategically place floor and table lamps around the room for ambience.

"THE KEY TO BEING A FANTASTIC ENTERTAINER
IS TO LOOK LIKE YOU ARE HAVING AN
AMAZING TIME—BECAUSE YOU REALLY *ARE*
ENJOYING YOURSELF, OF COURSE."

CREATE A DECIDED FLOW. Everything I do, from designing a collection to decorating a living room, calls for an easy energy. I don't care for anything that feels fussy or constricting in the end. The overall cadence carries over into my entertaining, too. A party should have a natural flow that you might have to gently nudge if it ambles off course. For instance, start everyone off with cocktails in one spacious room. Then, beckon them into another area—maybe a dining room—for supper, or outside for al fresco nibbles. By moving the party, even from one end of a room to another, you create some fluidity and energize people with a new setting. If my guests are all gridlocked in the kitchen during a party at our house, I'll motivate the crowd by saying "Everybody go outside and get some air!" Place candles, food, and fresh flowers wherever you want people to congregate. Otherwise, they may randomly stand in hallways.

INVIGORATE THE MOOD. Unfortunately, there is no foolproof recipe for inviting guests who always have excellent chemistry. And if people aren't mingling or having fun, I'll admit that I used to go into emotional cardiac arrest. How are you to know that two jewelry designers might not want to talk shop or that a usually gregarious couple will arrive sulking after an en route spat? When I detect a social lull among my guests, I do one of two things: recount an embarrassing personal moment that will loosen everyone up or whisper "Rodger, change the music." Believe me when I say that his music can make even the most uptight people shimmy a little in their seats.

RODGER'S PARTY PLAYLIST

Rachel and I both love a lot of the same music from the late sixties and early seventies. It's one of the interests we bonded over early on and I even convinced her to come to some Grateful Dead shows back in the day. If you come to a dinner party at our house, you're bound to hear these songs.

"Love Street," The Doors

"Lay Lady Lay," Bob Dylan

"All I Want Is You," U2

"Green Eyes," Coldplay

"Peggy-O," The Grateful Dead

"Landslide," Fleetwood Mac

"Everybody Hurts," R.E.M.

"Angie," The Rolling Stones

"Don't Tell Me," Madonna

"Get Together," The Youngbloods

SERVE LOW-KEY, UNCOMPLICATED FOOD. I won't try to dissuade you from adding a chilled gazpacho or a steaming bouillabaisse to the menu. But for me, the easiest way to feed a crowd without worry is with items that are best enjoyed at room temperature—especially at a casual dinner party. You'd be surprised how many different dishes fall into that category, from grilled rosemary chicken breast to sliced steak to poached salmon. When you are not tied to a menu that must be scheduled to accommodate temperatures, you're not hovering over a hot stove or oven and blotting at your face in between courses. Also, there is no urgency about eating. Your guests can dig in when they're ready and they don't feel compelled to end a fascinating conversation because the braised short ribs are getting cold. And everyone can come and go as they please.

DRESS FOR THE OCCASION

Part of the fun of playing hostess is deciding what to wear when you open the door. If your outfit includes a tiara at a dinner party, you set a silly and decadent tone. Similarly, your bare feet at a brunch immediately put everyone at ease—and might even encourage other guests to shuck off their shoes. For my own quick touch-ups, I tuck away a lipstick in my guest bathroom or kitchen so I can refresh my pout in seconds. My overall philosophy on what to wear when entertaining is that you should dress up and even take a few fashion risks. Wear that bold purple dress or the satin turban. Do a bright red lip. After all, everyone is looking at you—you should be stunning when you host. I love to finish my look with a statement piece like a choker, long chains, or bib necklace that infuses glamour. Of course, what you wear depends somewhat on the type of party. Here are some suggestions by occasion.

CHIC COCKTAILS. A jumpsuit is a cool and easy silhouette that can easily be amped up with sky-high heels and a few layered accessories.

CANDLELIT DINNER PARTY. Time for a little black dress that shows some décolletage with a gold choker that will reflect flickering tapers. If you're going to be popping up a lot to serve, avoid too many layers and fabric that might make you overheat.

CASUAL WEEKEND BRUNCH. Tailored dark denim with a fitted white tee and a boyfriend jacket looks effortlessly polished. I love to juxtapose the effect with a slightly messy topknot.

LATE-AFTERNOON BARBECUE. You can't go wrong with a bright, colorful maxi dress and gold gladiator flats. Keep in mind that heels and grass don't mix and that you may be sitting on a lawn, so anything super short could become X-rated. If you like a little extra height, opt for a comfortable wedge.

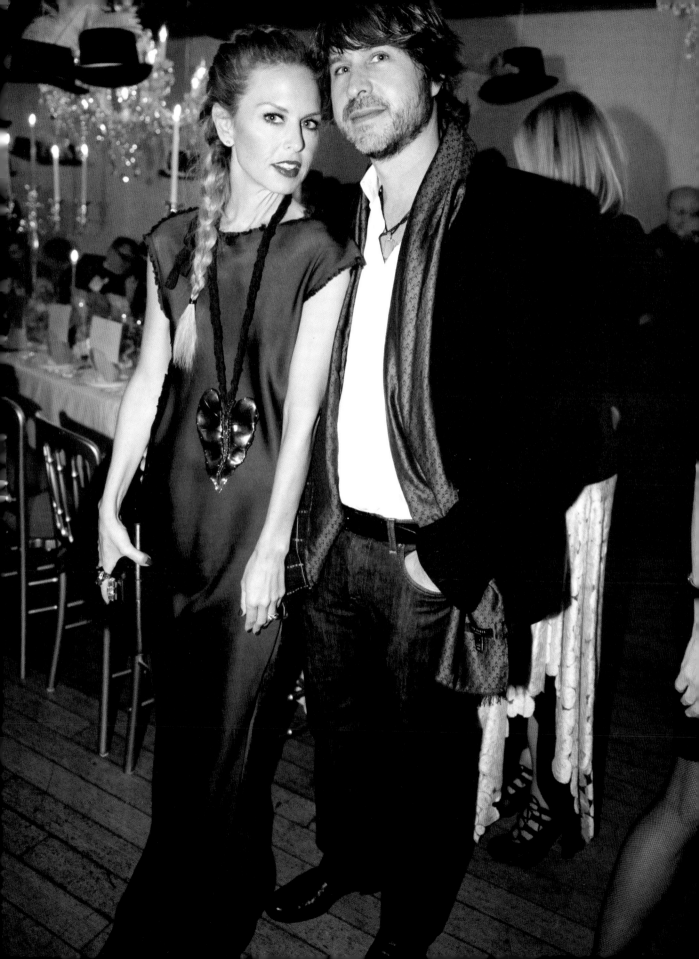

DIVIDE AND CONQUER

Have you ever attended an amazing party and wondered "How does she do it?" If she's savvy, she doesn't do it all alone. Delegating is imperative to pulling off a spectacular event—with your sanity intact. It could be that you divvy up the duties with your partner or a good friend. You might even consider cohosting a party; that way, you all share the work and cost and, in the end, bring new faces together.

Over the years, Rodger and I have developed and refined a system for entertaining that keeps us both busy and out of each other's path while we prep. He stocks the bar and does all the heavy lifting, from inching furniture around to fetching ice. I'm in charge of the cuisine, from shopping for ingredients to cooking or ordering and then setting the table.

We always create a timeline for an event, whether it's a Sunday supper for eight friends or a Studio 54–inspired dance party.

THREE WEEKS OUT: Think about your invitations, which can set the initial tone. I spend an hour or so on Paperless Post and gravitate toward a palette of white, black, and gold or tan. My wording—always in Century Gothic font, because it's timeless and strong—is typically minimal and to the point. Theme invites, with a grill for a barbecue or Champagne flutes for a celebration, are always fun.

TWO WEEKS OUT: Create a menu. Rodger and I start planning our dishes and a signature cocktail. We might serve festive sangria with blood oranges or a clear whiskey iced tea.

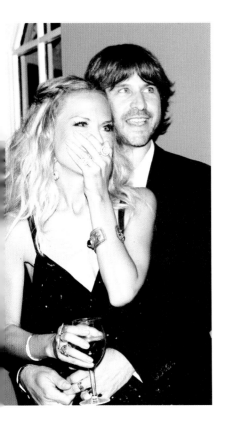

With Rodger at my birthday party, 2011

ONE WEEK OUT: Stock up on nonperishables. We shop for items such as tapered candles for the dining room table and spirits and mixers for the bar. If we are hosting a barbecue, we pick up plastic cutlery and recyclables. This is also a good time to assess seating and/or tables; look into rentals if necessary.

ONE TO TWO DAYS OUT: Time to double-check recipes and shop for essentials. We buy all the perishables—from charcuterie to fresh vegetables—within forty-eight hours of a party. Pick up any fresh flowers you'll want, and be sure you have appropriate vases. I also lay out my outfit at this point so I won't have to think about it on the day of the event.

THREE HOURS BEFOREHAND: Get glam. Though it might seem logical to wait until that last hour to shower and change into your outfit, something always comes up. I have learned to get ready earlier and then do the last minute tasks such as arranging cheese plates in my hostess wear.

ONE HOUR BEFOREHAND: Now that Rodger and I are cohosting with a toddler, it's not easy to control the schedule! Skyler runs around the house in a diaper while I chase him with his outfit, or put him to bed if we are entertaining in the later evening. I like to put platters out on the buffet table and pull out any last-minute items. We go through our checklist one last time and inevitably run to the local market for anything outstanding.

THIRTY MINUTES BEFOREHAND: Rodger deals with the beverages that need to be chilled and then puts on the music. I light candles. We always strive to be done with prep about a half hour before guests arrive. That way, we can relax and have a chill moment together before the doorbell rings.

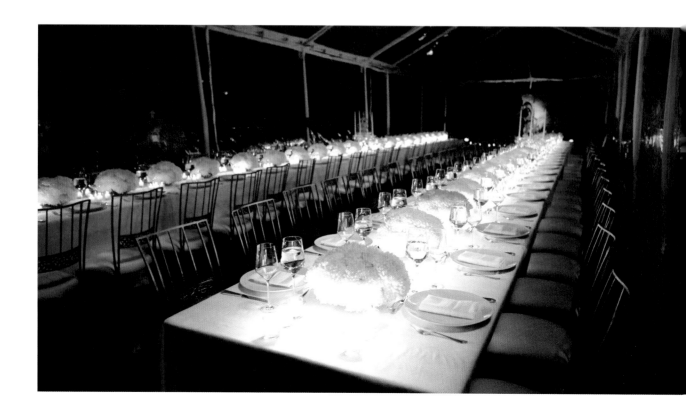

Left and right: The décor at my non-traditional baby shower, hosted by Pamela Skaist-Levy. Center: A formal table setting.

A TABLE IS A RUNWAY

By now, you might have already gathered that our décor aesthetic is rooted in a soft, neutral palette. Not shockingly, the same goes for my take on a beautifully set dinner table. I like a muted palette here, because it reminds me of a fashion runway. The vivid colors and varied textures of food and bright décor accents pop on this canvas. Most of my dishes are white; my Tiffany wedding china bears only a discreet platinum edge. A classic border on a plate, whether it's chevron or chain links, makes an interesting side note to the meal. My mom taught me to sometimes use chargers as dinner plates. That way, everyone has enough room on their dishes to try everything on the table. On occasion, though, I love to mix up my plates and juxtapose formal with casual accents. Simple stemware looks cool next to ornate china; modern flatware adds some edge to antique patterned dishes. Colored or clear glass bowls inject a little whimsy to a table, too. My collection of oversized square simple white dinner plates are unexpected and look graphic and bold.

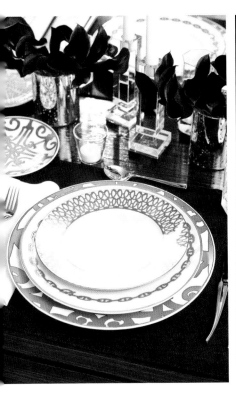

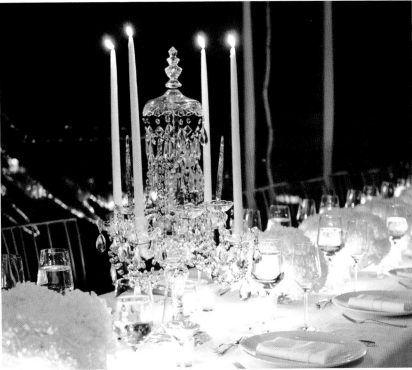

If I want to create a more formal and elegant setting, I break out the silverware, occasion glasses, soup bowls, and bread plates. A few easy rules for setup: Linens should be placed on the center of the plate or folded and to the left. Plates should be layered according to use, e.g., the first-course plate—be it a salad or soup—will rest on top. A bread plate goes above the forks, which are to the left of the plate. Forks start at the outside according to use, so have a salad fork to the left of the main utensil. The knife sits to the right of the plate, with the blade facing inward. Finally, glasses go above the knife, starting with water and then wine stems.

We have an immense zebra wood rectangular table that seats twelve, but it was custom-made to be extra wide. I like an expanse of space, because I often serve meals family style. If I am going to put out huge bouquets of fresh-cut flowers—such as peeled back roses made famous by my favorite floral designer, Eric Buterbaugh—and giant serving platters of delicious food, I can't bear a cramped, cluttered table. A few dramatic candelabras or a row of votives can take up precious real estate on a table. But be as creative with your table as you are with your personal style. Bright neon fruit like lemons or limes pop in a glass cylinder vase or even artfully scattered down the center of the table. Rosemary or lavender tied around a napkin or centered on a plate always looks romantic.

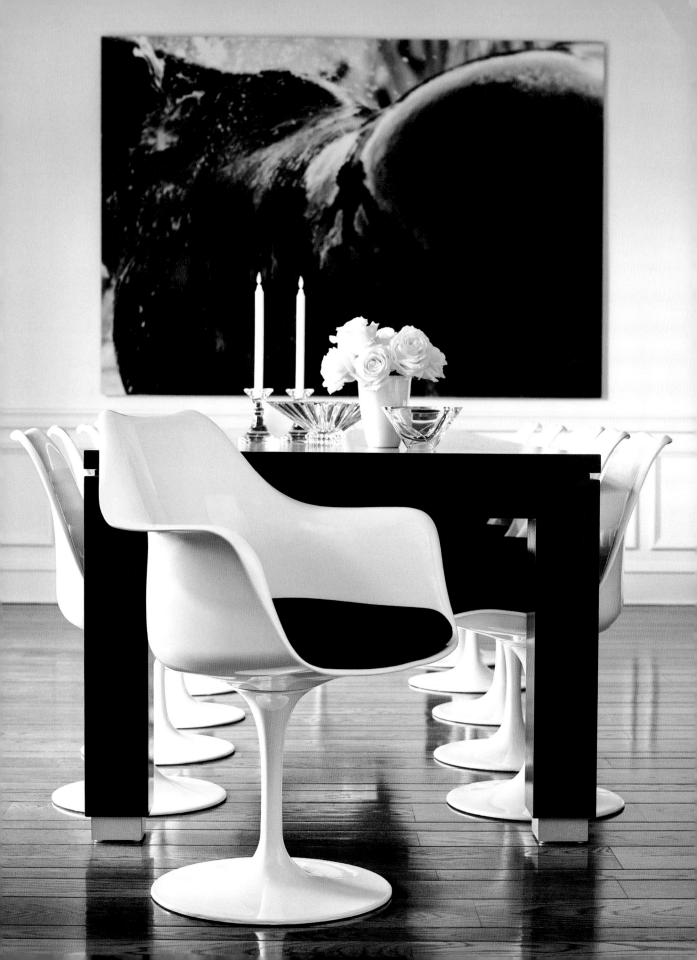

DRAMATIC BLOOMS

Flowers are one of my favorite indulgences for entertaining, but they don't always cooperate. I'm partial to these temperamental ones in monochromatic single varietal bunches, so I know how to care for them.

HYDRANGEAS:
These clouds of blossoms are hearty and gorgeous, but can also wilt suddenly. Place stems in very hot water for 30 seconds if flowers droop—they should perk up and stay fresh for up to five more days.

PHALAENOPSIS ORCHIDS:
I love that these exotic plants are dramatic, yet affordable. You can even buy them at some grocery stores. They bloom only once or twice a year, but their flowers last up to three months if you add three ice cubes to the container per week and keep them out of direct sunlight.

CALLA LILIES:
Fluted like Champagne glasses, these graceful flowers tend to bend at their stems in the same direction. I'm crazy for the "black" variety, which are actually a deep, rich red. In arranging them, be gentle so as to avoid bruising.

PEONIES:
High season for these spectacular round blooms is spring—sadly, they're scarce in winter. If the buds won't open, place them in warm water and on a sunny ledge.

TULIPS:
Keep these fragile slender-stemmed blooms away from direct sunlight and heating vents. You can add a penny or two to the water to make them last a few days longer.

Peeled back roses by Eric Buterbaugh

For seating, we have a dozen white fiberglass Eero Saarinen tulip swivel chairs designed for Knoll back in the mid 1950s. Each one, with its fluted lines and pedestal base, looks like a piece of sculpture. The architect and designer once said that he created the one-legged chair to minimize clutter—a man after my own heart. It's also easy to be able to turn to talk intimately with someone on your left or right.

I rarely assign seating because I trust that my guests are all outgoing and inclusive. But if you invite a group of people who don't know each other at all and feel anxious about it, think ahead and use cute place cards to put together people who have common interests. That way, you won't have

Opposite: The dining room

to worry about hovering and igniting conversations all night. Some hosts don't like to let couples sit next to each other—but not me. I understand that my dinner party might be the only time they have together all day or even all weekend. When it comes to conversation, I always encourage my guests to tell personal stories and talk about current events. If you're seated next to someone you don't know at a dinner, a smart, original inquiry always ignites a dialogue. It can also be a lively icebreaker for a hostess to throw out to the table between courses. My only forbidden topic? Politics. People get extremely heated over hot-button issues—especially after a few glasses of wine—and suddenly, half the table could be heading out the door.

SCENTS AND SENSIBILITY

Fragrance is an accessory for your home and it always impacts the ambience of a party. Perfumed candles do double duty, but be sure the scent isn't too overpowering. The same rule applies to room sprays and artfully placed potpourri. You can have different fragrances from room to room, reserving a spicy, sensual fragrance for the cocktails area and a floral one for the bathroom. My favorites?

AMBER:
Spicy, exotic, warm notes make the perfect olfactory palette for a get-together on a cold night. Fantastic for an Oscar party.

FIG:
I adore the subtly sweet earthiness of this fragrance with its milky accents. Keep one candle flickering in the foyer to set the tone for a dinner party.

LAVENDER:
No matter the occasion, this gentle herbal scent always soothes the scene and helps people relax. I love it for daytime events.

TUBEROSE:
This highly intoxicating floral feels romantic and mysterious—it's also known for its aphrodisiac properties, making it the perfect redolence for a sexy cocktail party.

SANDALWOOD:
It's no surprise that Tom Ford has a fragrance called Santal Blush. Super sensual with a strong woodsy finish, it's the ideal backdrop for a first date at the house or romantic night in.

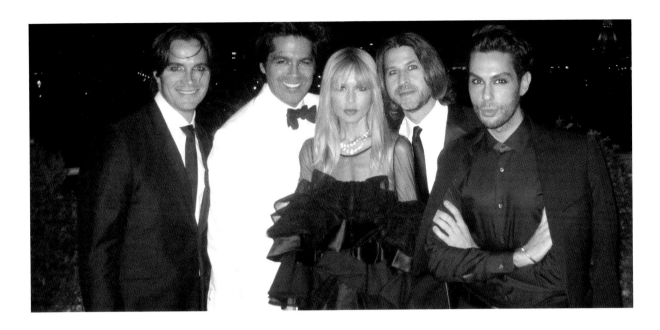

*With friends attending
Carine Roitfeld's "Black Tie,
Smoky Eye" event in Paris*

ATTIRE: BLACK-TIE, SMOKY EYE

Los Angeles might be the epicenter of unfathomable dress codes. I have seen invitations that call for bizarre attires like "denim dazzle" (two words that should never collide, in my opinion) and "corporate elegant." Suggested party attire should never confuse guests or, worse, force them to panic and spend a week's pay on an elaborate costume or a cocktail dress in a specific hue like pale lemon or Vreeland red.

Instead, take a cue from my style icon Carine Roitfeld, former editor-in-chief of French *Vogue* and now the global fashion director at *Harper's Bazaar*. In Paris, during Fashion Week fall 2012, she hosted a blowout party called Le Bal with a "black tie, smoky eye" dress code. What I loved about this particular directive is that everybody could kohl their eyes and raid their closets for a stunning getup—it didn't require any additional hassle or effort. Rodger even played along and borrowed my eyeliner!

When Rodger and I got married at the Rainbow Room in New York in 1998, our wedding was a black-tie affair—even though we walked down the aisle to the Grateful Dead's iconic anthem, "Truckin'." (My dad and I danced to Stevie Nicks's "Landslide," a favorite song of mine.) But other than that occasion, I can't think of a time I asked my guests to style themselves a certain way. I'm not averse to sensible theme parties or dress codes at all; rather, I just appreciate my friends' collective and individual style so much that I let them handle their own attire.

TIMING IS EVERYTHING

I try to be on time, if not early, for everything—especially when I am in New York, where you can set your watch by certain people. In Los Angeles, punctuality is considered a lost art, but I still think it's a sign of respect to show up at an appointed time. When people have to wait for you, they can't help but feel you assume their time isn't valuable. That's never a solid foundation for any relationship—personal *or* professional.

When I throw a dinner party, I typically call for cocktails an hour or so earlier than the time we sit down to eat. That gives everyone a cushion for when to arrive—but still, some people always seem to show up during dessert. At the age of eighty-six, Coco Chanel complained in an interview that people were sauntering into dinner parties two hours late in Paris; she called it vulgar. Coco would go insane if she lived in L.A.!

There is, however, a social drawback to being punctual: Sometimes you get to an event before the room fills. Walking into a party and not seeing any familiar faces used to give me a panic attack. Seriously, I would exit as soon as I politely could. But after years of attending luncheons and cocktail parties and lavish European-style business dinners, I have learned that it's better to get to a party when it's already in full swing and then leave just after the party has peaked. (Plus, I now devote my early evening to feeding my son and tucking him in before I go out.) I always ask ahead for the nod to bring a guest along so I can be sure I will know at least one person there, but sometimes, a plus one is impossible and you have to respect that request. Besides, flying solo is a great opportunity to socialize outside your comfort zone.

When you're out alone, look for a familiar face—even if you have met a person only once—and strike up a conversation. You can even be honest and admit you don't know anyone else and plan to shadow him or her. Another idea is to seek out the host and insist on helping out, whether that's opening a bottle of wine or putting out a platter. It's a great way to meet other guests, as the host will be greeting people as they arrive and make introductions. People will flock to where there is food and drink, so try stationing yourself there. Or, you can try to flatter a guest who looks interesting. A well-aimed compliment will endear you to someone every time—but be sure it's sincere. Look for the person wearing an amazing dress or killer jewelry and ask about it. If you're just not feeling super out-going, plan to arrive at the end of the cocktail hour or mingling portion of an event. That way, you can take your place at the table and instantly have someone to talk to on either side.

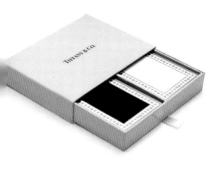

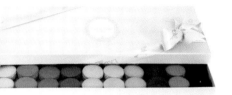

GIVING AND RECEIVING

Whenever I entertain, I always instruct my guests not to bring anything at all. It's a good policy, because it takes the pressure off people to find the perfect token of thanks. Still, many of my friends arrive with *something*. In my opinion, the best hostess gifts are ones that can be enjoyed later. For instance, I will never thrust a layer cake or bouquet of fresh flowers into the hands of the host, because either offering requires immediate attention and might not complement what she or he had planned. Instead, a box of exotic chocolate truffles or a set of designer playing cards tops my list.

Sometimes, Rodger and I will give our host a classic game such as Monopoly or Scrabble as a gift. (After a few cocktails, board games can get very, very interesting.) I'm also partial to gorgeous coasters, elegant serving trays, and oversized glossy fashion or photography books like *Halston: An American Original* or *Poolside with Slim Aarons*. A box of gold embossed note cards is a thoughtful token, too. (Just insist that the host needn't use one as a thank-you note to you!) A cute or funny apron can be an unexpected and functional offering. But at the end of the day, you can never go wrong with an incredibly great bottle of wine or Champagne. Put it in a gold or silver wine sleeve with a little note or just tie on a ribbon to personalize it.

A recent study revealed that more than half the country feels fine about regifting. That's great, but I'm not one of them. I support recycling, but I think it's bad karma to pass along a present someone gave to me. I will, however, pay forward a sweater or scarf or accessory that doesn't work for me. I always preface it with "Someone gave this to me, but I can't use it. It's more you than me." That way, it's clear that I am regifting.

Top: A set of playing cards by Tiffany & Co. Bottom: Macaroons by La Durée.

Next spread: A selection of keepsake thank-you notes

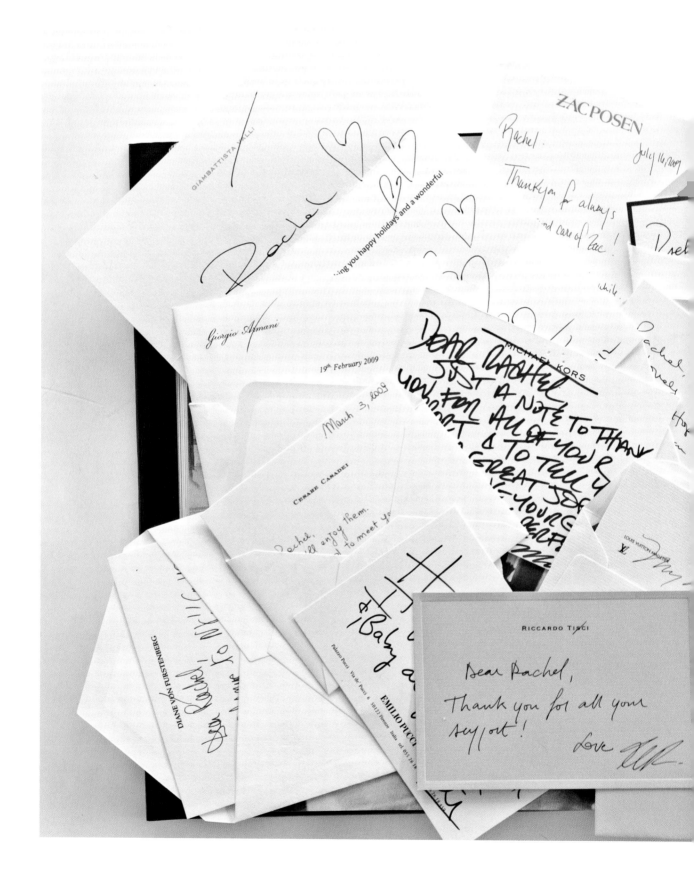

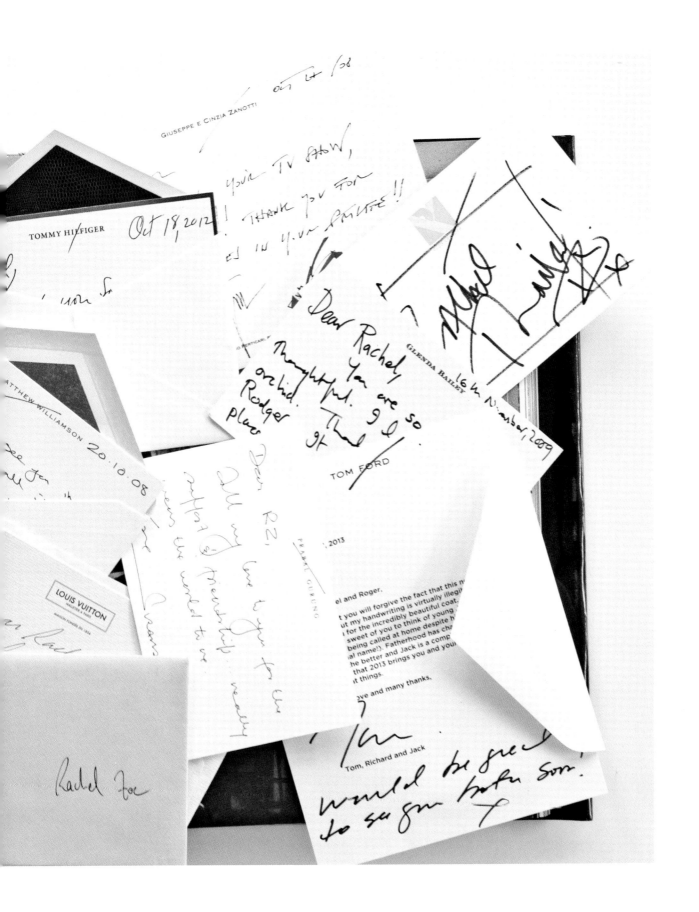

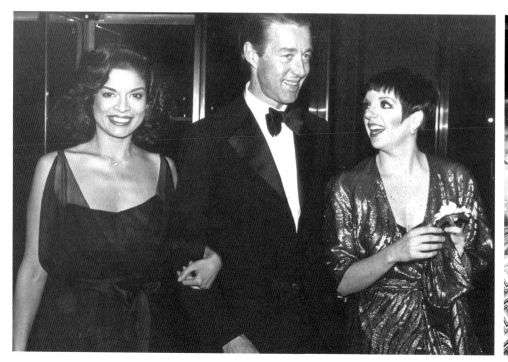
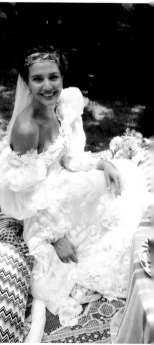

*Left: Bianca Jagger,
Halston, and Liza Minnelli.
Right: Margherita Missoni
on her wedding day.*

MERCI IN THE NEW MILLENNIUM

Never underestimate the value of a thank-you. In an ideal world, I would be known for my handwritten notes of appreciation on embossed stationery with tissue paper–lined envelopes. To me, they are incredibly thoughtful and personal, and make a distinctive keepsake. I keep a collection of letters and notes I have received from friends, designers, and clients in a special box just because I treasure them. The paper stock is creamy and thick and the scrawled messages are sometimes witty and sly. They feel like pieces of art.

"NEVER UNDERESTIMATE THE VALUE OF A THANK-YOU."

But my own go-to for gratitude is electronic. It's not only better for the environment, but I can pen a sincere thank-you anywhere, whether I'm waiting for a dinner date or sitting in an airport. Within forty-eight hours of receiving a gift or attending a dinner, I make a point to send an e-mail with a heartfelt message. Because e-thanks can seem impersonal, it's important to call out something specific. I might gush about the design of a piece of jewelry someone has given to me or mention how much I loved discussing the agony of getting my son to nap over lunch. I draw the line at thank-you texts, though. Seven characters of gratitude just doesn't cut it.

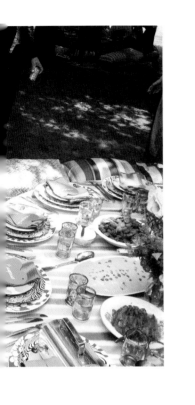

INFORMAL, BUT UNFORGETTABLE

Fashion people love any excuse to wear beautiful clothes. Look back at photos from Studio 54's heyday and you'll spot Halston, in a white silk scarf, laughing uproariously on the arm of Liza Minnelli.

Or a tuxedoed and bespectacled Yves Saint Laurent doing a social lap with the divine Catherine Deneuve. Don't get me started again on how much I long to have lived in the seventies and hit the scene at the venerable hot spot. That whole moment epitomizes this unforced glamour and verve to me. There was an ease to the way people entertained and enjoyed themselves.

Of course, the modern-day fashion world knows how to celebrate, too. And in my twenty years in the business so far, I have been lucky enough to attend dozens upon dozens of over-the-top, fantastic events. Valentino's forty-fifth anniversary extravaganza comes to mind: a black-tie party on the grounds of the Villa Borghese with aerialist ballerinas pirouetting in front of the Colosseum. I must have gasped a dozen times during the thirty-six-hour event!

Casual gatherings can be just as impressive. Some of my favorite stylish entertainers and dear friends have managed to make low-key get-togethers feel equally special, even opulent, in an organic way. The Missoni family, for instance, hosts weekends in Italy with kids frolicking in and out of their villa, amid mismatched plates and all sorts of eclectic cuisines.

Diane von Furstenberg invites her dear friends over to her Paris apartment to sit around in a circle on overstuffed ethnic floor pillows. The supremely witty Marc Jacobs prefers a close-knit dinner party of four or six guests who wouldn't ordinarily come together; he loves to choreograph the conversation of a disparate group. Stella McCartney inspires me because she adheres to her lifelong activist ideals when she throws a party. The menu is always vegan and delicious. Above all, the takeaway is to remember that it's all about the company you keep and your own style of entertaining. No matter what you serve or how you set a table, your guests will always have an amazing time if you relax, be yourself, and have fun, too.

CHAPTER 8

GOING PLACES

Travel was a huge part of my childhood. My parents strongly believed that seeing other parts of the world and learning about the cultures of other countries made a person more well rounded and savvier about life. I couldn't agree more. When I was twelve, they took my sister and me on an unforgettable vacation to Italy. I can still remember walking around Venice, astounded by the beauty of the city. On this particular trip, I also fell hard for chic European style and discovered my obsession with fashion. I noticed how the women relied on simple, well-cut silhouettes, luxurious fabrics, and dramatic accessories to look elegant. Still, whenever I travel, I take note of the local style and nuances. I also make a mental note of the colors and shapes of the landscapes. When I sit down to conceptualize a collection, I envision those women and their surroundings. It's hardly shocking that many of my style icons are European.

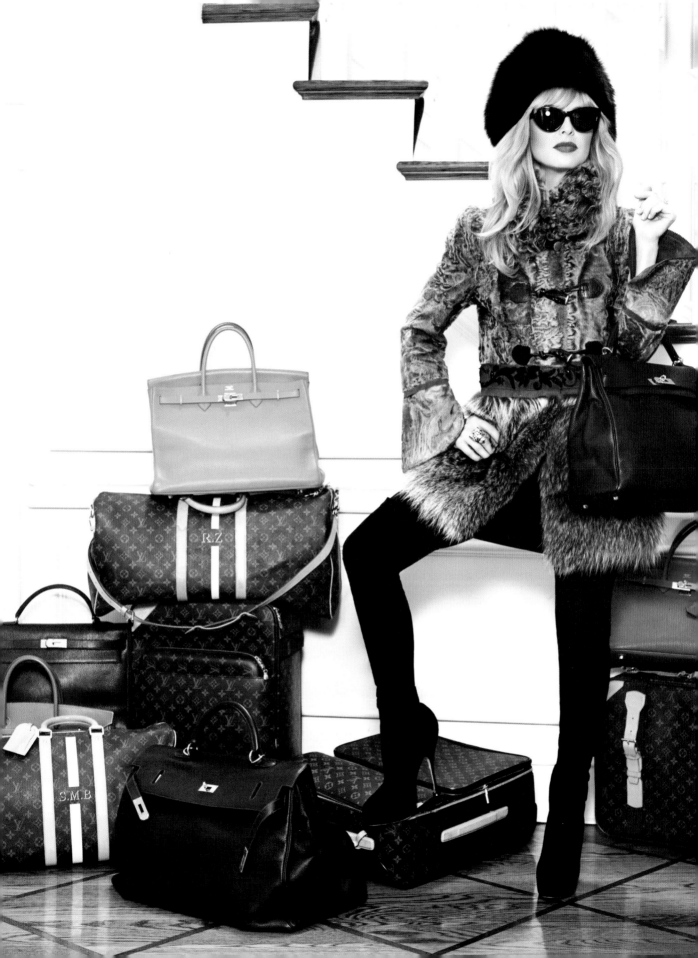

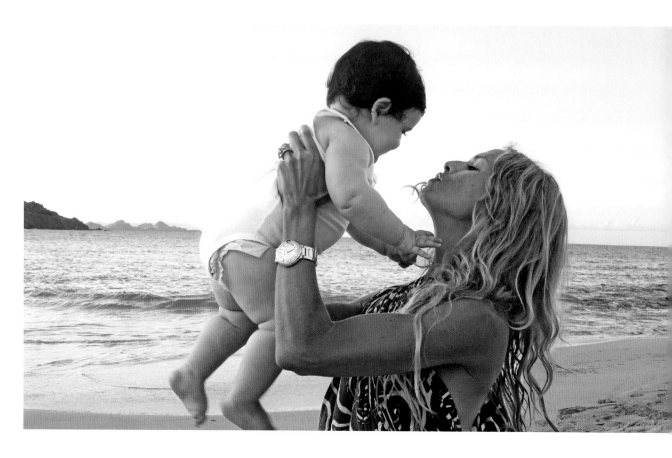

With Skyler in Saint Bart's

I even save all my old passports and the colorful currencies from different countries. Rodger and I have this dream to rent a villa for a month on the Amalfi Coast of Italy or in Tuscany when Skyler gets a little older. In my fantasy, I see us walking into the nearby little village to buy fresh pasta, Parmesan, a bottle of Pinot Grigio, and a loaf of bread for dinner. We will learn some Italian while Skyler makes new friends. Unlike my breathless and busy trips to Paris, our European family hiatus will be snail-paced, quiet, and a bit like a Bertolucci film—until the pipes burst in our eighteenth century villa, of course.

It's as important to take do-nothing vacations as it is to soak up culture. Our lives are overscheduled enough. You shouldn't underestimate the value of spending one day being lazy. My MO when we head to Saint Bart's every year is to do absolutely nothing but gaze out at the ocean, play with Skyler in the sand, and meet up with friends for casual dinners. I recharge while I'm there and come back to work feeling refreshed and even inspired by the vivid hues of a dramatic sunset or the way a light fabric billows in an afternoon breeze.

PACK LIKE A PRO

Every year, I take at least two major trips. In August, it's off to New York and then Europe for almost six weeks of runway shows, including my own shows and events during fashion season. And at the end of the year, it's the getaway to Saint Bart's. The first is not an easy pack, as I'm in New York when we show the collection in early fall and the weather can be unpredictable—think humid and sunny one morning and a dreary downpour an hour later. Then, I head to Paris, London, and Milan, where I might need a coat and lots of cold weather accessories. Since I'm jet-setting through time zones and different climates, I have learned to begin organizing my wardrobe weeks ahead of time. Saint Bart's—where I mostly live in caftans, sarongs, and wide-brimmed hats—calls for some thought about day-to-day looks and evening outfits. Last-minute packing always results in overdoing it—just ask Rodger. Now, I have a tried-and-true timeline for packing smart, no matter the destination:

TWO WEEKS OUT: I like to create an "outfit itinerary" after looking at the schedule of my trip, especially with business travel. Note the time and nature of each event and then lay out a potential look—including accessories—for that occasion. I might mark down velvet tuxedo with booties for an afternoon meeting with a retailer or a printed maxi dress, leather jacket, and platform wedges for a cocktail party. If you notice any gaps, you have plenty of time to find new pieces before you go. And you can always ask friends to fill in the blanks with a borrowed evening clutch or a cashmere scarf.

This is also a good time to set aside pieces that need to be dry-cleaned or shoes that could use a new heel or sole. The same goes for accessories—check clasps on necklaces or bracelets and make sure that all the earrings you plan to pack are in pairs. I always photograph my options with my phone so I have an easy-to-access reference guide.

If you're taking a lengthy trip or packing beyond what you can manage at the airport, consider shipping items ahead of time. By planning a few weeks in advance, you can send a suitcase across the country via FedEx Ground and pay about sixty-five dollars for a fifty-pound bag that arrives in four business days; but overnight service runs closer to three hundred dollars.

ONE WEEK OUT: Check the weather report for any unexpected climate changes and alter your outfit lineup accordingly. Review the photos of your looks if you took them, and make notes on any necessary tweaks. I always swap out a few pieces or experiment with different accessories—it's the stylist in me. If you purchased a new pair of shoes for the trip, wear them for an entire day to break them in and to ensure that they are comfortable. There is nothing worse than blisters on a vacation!

Refill any prescriptions that may be low and assess all your beauty products to be sure that you won't run out of moisturizer or foundation while away. Pick up three-ounce travel bottles to transfer liquids for carry-on use. I like to schedule a manicure, pedicure, and blowout for the day or so before I travel. I always pick up my chosen nail polishes so I will have them handy for on-the-go touch-ups. Who hasn't chipped a nail at the airport?

THREE DAYS OUT: I call ahead to the hotel to request extra hangers. You can also ask if they offer steamers to guests. (If not, put a handheld one aside to pack.) Contact your credit card companies to alert them of your trip—especially when traveling overseas—so that none of your charges will be declined. Arrange to have your mail handled and suspend your newspaper subscription if need be.

TWO DAYS OUT: Finalize your outfits and put all shoes, clothes, and accessories aside. As a stylist, this is what I call the "big edit." Make sure your pieces are truly versatile: a cool leather jacket and a sleek black dress are items you can accessorize a few different ways. Look at your shoe picks through the same prism: Can you wear that pair of suede over-the-knee boots with a few outfits? Do you really need two pairs of black pumps? I would rather overpack accessories like scarves, hats, bags, and statement jewelry. Not only do these accents take up less space, but they also complete your signature style. At this point, also load up with reading material and make a mellow playlist for the flight.

THE DAY BEFORE: Pack! I have learned not to wait until the day of a trip to organize my suitcase. Packing your suitcase the day before allows you to make last-minute tweaks and substitutions. My method is to use the dust bags that come with handbags to separate all my essentials. Undergarments go in one, scarves in another; same with T-shirts and tights. Shoes, of course, go in their own dust bags as well. (Any

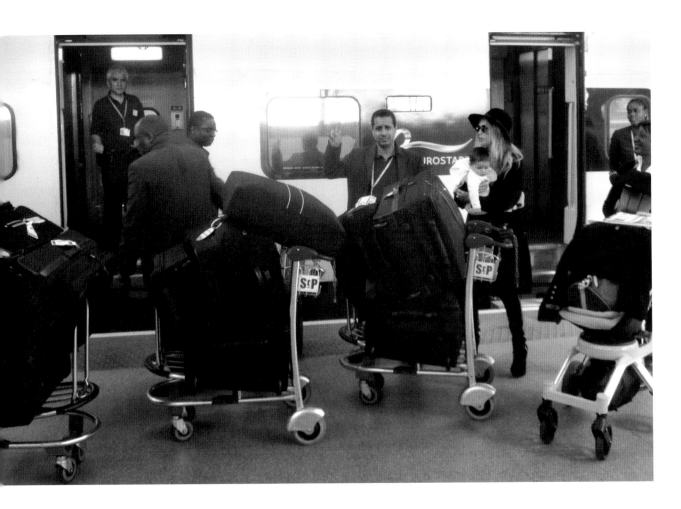

Arriving in Paris with Skyler and lots of luggage

soft pouches will work.) I place all the heaviest items like bags, shoes, and belts in the bottom and then layer clothes on hangers on top. My sequined pieces, silks, and any other fragile garments stay in dry cleaner bags to prevent any snags or pulls.

THE DAY OF: Set aside at least thirty minutes more than you think you will need to get out the door—there are always a few stray things to do, and you don't want to panic about missing a flight. Stow certain last-minute carry-on items such as a cell phone charger and any snacks for the plane. Your travel outfit could profoundly affect your comfort over a span of hours, so be sure to wear clothes that won't constrict you. I typically choose roomy, even slouchy pieces like a sweater dress or leggings with a jersey tee and duster. You won't catch me in any color but black, which can camouflage both stains and wrinkles. My secret weapon is an over-the-knee boot that ties the whole ensemble together.

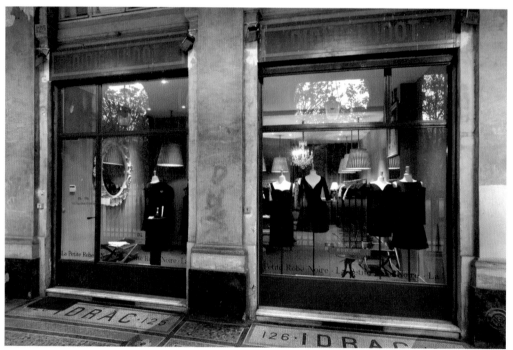
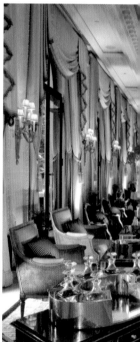

Left: Didier Ludot, Paris.
Right: Four Seasons
Hotel George V, Paris.

J'ADORE PARIS

Every visit to Paris feels like the very first one—even though I have been there almost forty times. I always see something new in the architecture, the museums, the cafés, or even the little shops on the side streets. Then, there are the people. They look so poised and stylish. Even the Parisian children carry themselves with elegance. I swear to you, the babies are born inherently chic over there. I get more inspired in Paris than in any other city in the world.

Because I have a finite amount of time to visit the boutiques and flea markets, I become anxious to shop as soon as I arrive. A word of advice: If you fall in love with a dress, a painting, or a purse while traveling, buy it. First of all, that item will always remind you of your trip and spur a little nostalgia. Second, it's likely you won't be able to find it stateside—and there's nothing worse than retail regret. (Rodger and I have shipped home vintage lamps from Paris and a rug from Saint Bart's for that reason!) You don't want to think of Rome as the place where you *didn't* buy those amazing equestrian boots.

In Paris, I usually hit my favorite vintage shops first. I love a boutique in the Saint Germain called Les 3 Marches de Catherine B. It's like going

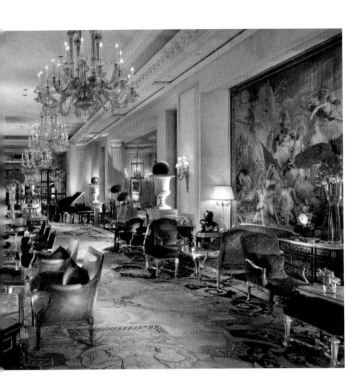

to a museum to shop, completely stocked with pristine Chanel pieces. Browsing vintage haute couture at the gorgeous emporium Didier Ludot in the gardens of the Palais Royal is a must, too. If I'm there over the weekend, I always go to the big antique flea market called Les Puces de Saint-Ouen, where you can find everything from a vintage Rolex to the most incredible deco light fixture.

Where to stay? I like to get to know at least one neighborhood of a foreign city as much as possible, so I make it a point to pick hotels in a specific area whenever I visit. That way, you can stake out your favorite café and visit every morning for a coffee or at sunset for a glass of wine. Pretty soon, the owner starts to recognize you and smiles or winks when you walk in; maybe his little French bulldog trots over, too. You can feel like a local even when you're away from home. I adore the Four Seasons Hotel George V off the Champs-Elysées and near avenue Montaigne. There are the most fabulous flower installations by the brilliant Jeff Leatham that he changes out almost every day and many of the rooms have beautiful terraces.

With Marc Jacobs at his home in Paris

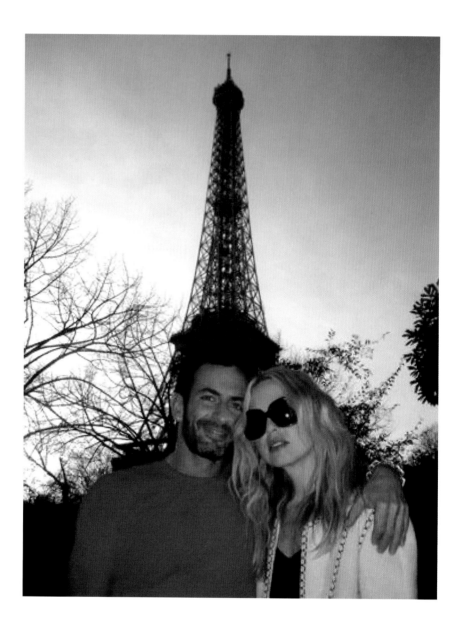

The courtyard at Hôtel Costes on rue Saint-Honoré is where I eat lunch almost every day during Paris Fashion Week. You literally see every designer there—I used to spot Yves Saint Laurent eating in the corner with his partner. I would shake with excitement just catching a glimpse of him! When I'm not people watching, I love to visit the Louvre, and the Opéra National de Paris, where Stella McCartney has shown her collections in the past few years, is a beautiful building, too. It was built in the 1600s by Louis XIV, so it's incredibly opulent and over the top.

"EVERY VISIT TO PARIS FEELS LIKE THE VERY FIRST ONE."

If I'm taking a trip to somewhere I don't know quite as well, I typically forgo travel books for word-of-mouth suggestions from friends. That way, your itinerary is more personal. A few weeks before a vacation, I e-mail friends who I know have visited my planned destination and ask for their favorite cafés, secret beaches, and vintage or antique stores. Sometimes, I am more specific and ask what the best spot is to catch a breathtaking sunset, or say "Tell me about the flea market where you got that amazing vintage clutch." I rely on this method of planning so heavily that I asked some of my most stylish and well-traveled friends to contribute insight on their favorite places in the world—from London to Buenos Aires. Their suggestions make me want to pack a bag and go!

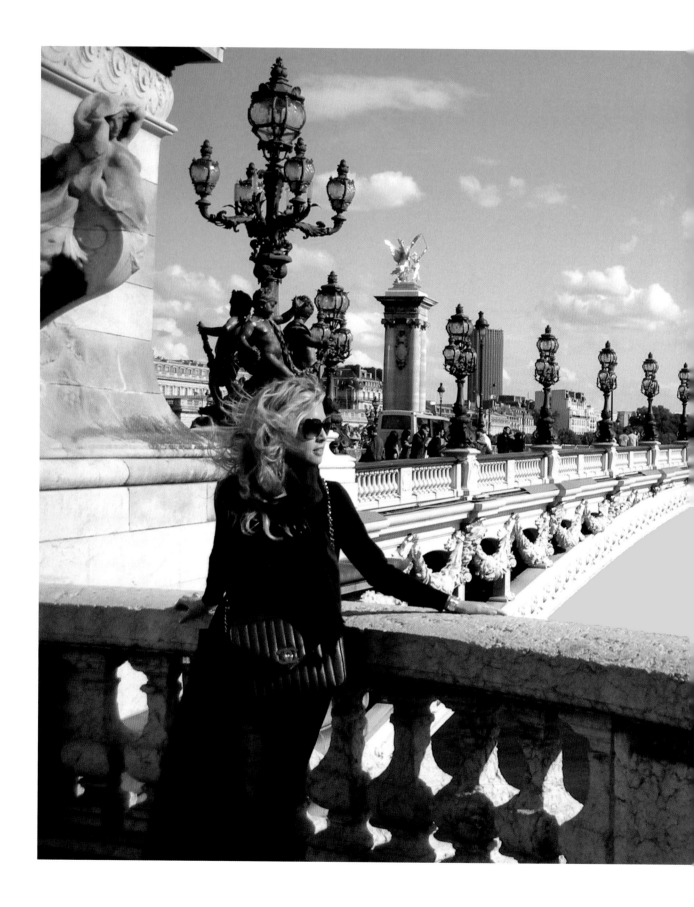

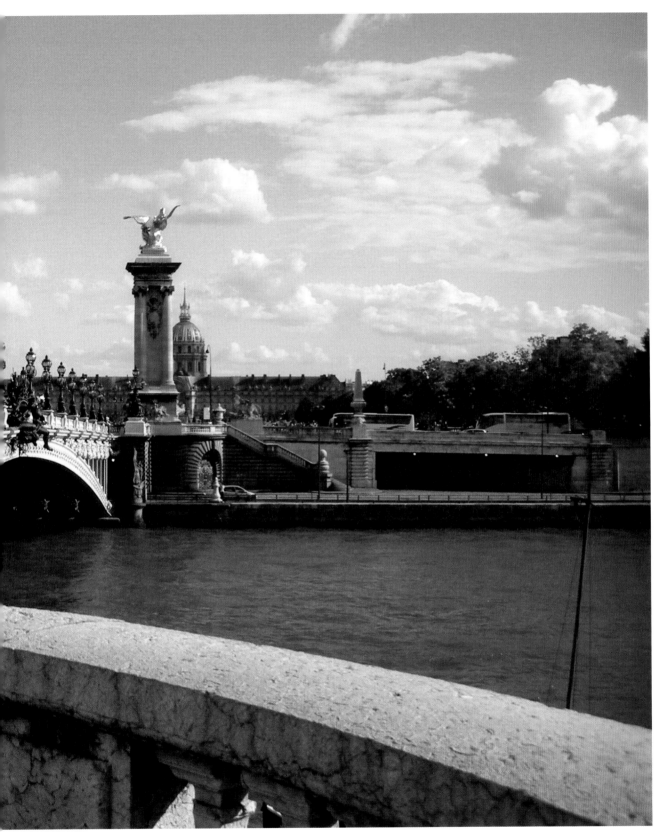

In Paris

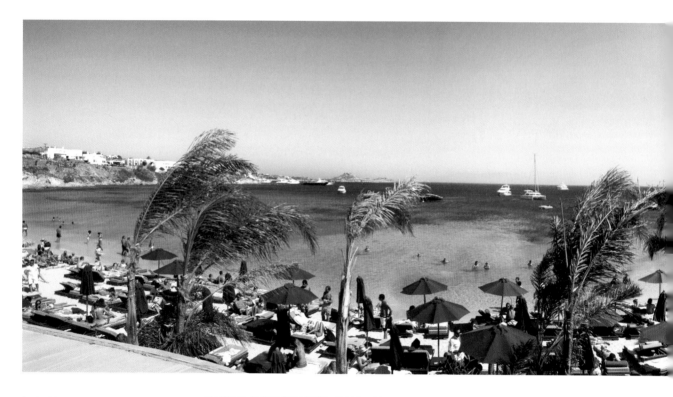

Left: Nammos restaurant, Mykonos. Right: The Cotton House hotel, Mustique.

SHOE DESIGNER BRIAN ATWOOD ON MYKONOS

In Mykonos, the energy, the light, and the sea are all intoxicating. It's a traveler's utopia, unlike anywhere else in the world. There is a sensuality about the people and the island and the food that has me hooked. Kiki's, a taverna with no electricity situated under a tree, has the best octopus I've ever eaten. Everybody waits for a table—there are no reservations. The beachside restaurant Nammos is the place to see and be seen. Arrive preferably by yacht and plan to dance on tables by the end of your meal. The best hotel is the Belvedere, but I have rented the same villa for the past several years.

Staying in a home away from it all makes my time in Mykonos more relaxing and intimate. Usually the house is packed with ten to fifteen of my family members and friends. We often go to Kapari Beach—it's private, has a chic crowd, and even some nudity!

You can't leave Mykonos without an evil eye souvenir. You can find a colorful multi-wrap bracelet for two euros, or really high-end handmade pieces that are exquisite. ■

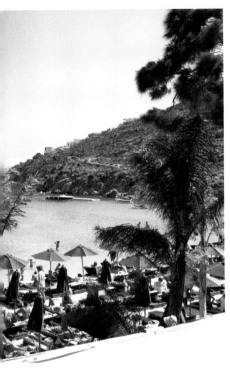

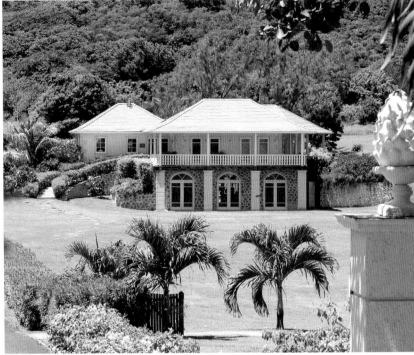

FASHION DESIGNER MATTHEW WILLIAMSON ON MUSTIQUE

The remote private island of Mustique is an idyllic paradise, with endless stretches of white sand, turquoise waters, and lush greenery. Its isolated nature is a huge part of its appeal. When I'm feeling social, I go to Basil's Bar, which is an institution that serves impeccably fresh fish and seafood. They do an amazing lime daiquiri, too.

I like to stay at the Cotton House hotel, which has beautiful rooms and exceptional service—they host a cocktail party for the island's inhabitants each week. If I have an hour to kill, I might take a boat and explore some of the secluded bays and coves around the island. The waters around Mustique are full of beautiful reefs and tropical fish. It's a wonderful aquarium! ■

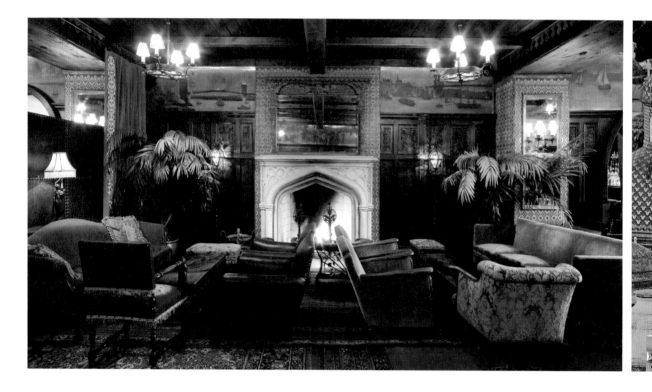

Left: The Bowery Hotel,
New York. Right: Old
district of Recoleta,
Buenos Aires.

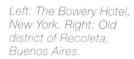

CALVIN KLEIN DESIGNER FRANCISCO COSTA ON NEW YORK CITY

I love the forwardness and constant energy of New York—its adrenaline, fresh ideas, and driven people are all inspiring. Because of the vertical nature of the city's architecture, you're always looking up. The High Line is the perfect place to go for a walk and escape. This elevated public park provides the best of both worlds, combining the city with its natural surroundings.

When I am down on the Lower East Side, I enjoy eating at The Fat Radish and visiting all the modern galleries, like Lisa Cooley and Orchard Windows Gallery. Casa in the West Village has the most delicious, authentic Brazilian food in New York City—their okra and chicken stew always remind me of home.

You can't go wrong staying at The Carlyle, because it is super chic, but if you are looking for something more downtown, then The Bowery Hotel is a cool option. ■

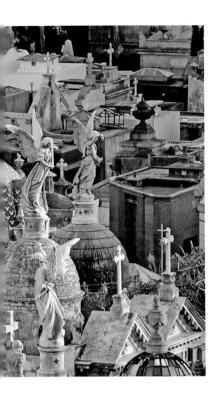

POLO PLAYER NACHO FIGUERAS ON BUENOS AIRES

Buenos Aires is known as the Paris of South America because of its European design, dating back to the beginning of the twentieth century.

Palermo Viejo is an older neighborhood that's great for discovering hip restaurants and small boutiques. I love the restaurants Sucre, La Panaderia de Pablo, and an amazing little coffee shop called I Love Café in the Recoleta area. If you want to sound like a local, order a *fernet con Coca,* an herbal Italian liquor mixed with Coca-Cola.

On a lazy afternoon, I like to walk around the old district of Recoleta, a beautiful historic neighborhood that is one of the highest points of the city. Before you leave Buenos Aires, you must pick up a beautiful handcrafted maté, which is a silver-trimmed calabash gourd used for drinking tea from the leaves of yerba maté. It comes with a silver straw called a *bombilla.* ∎

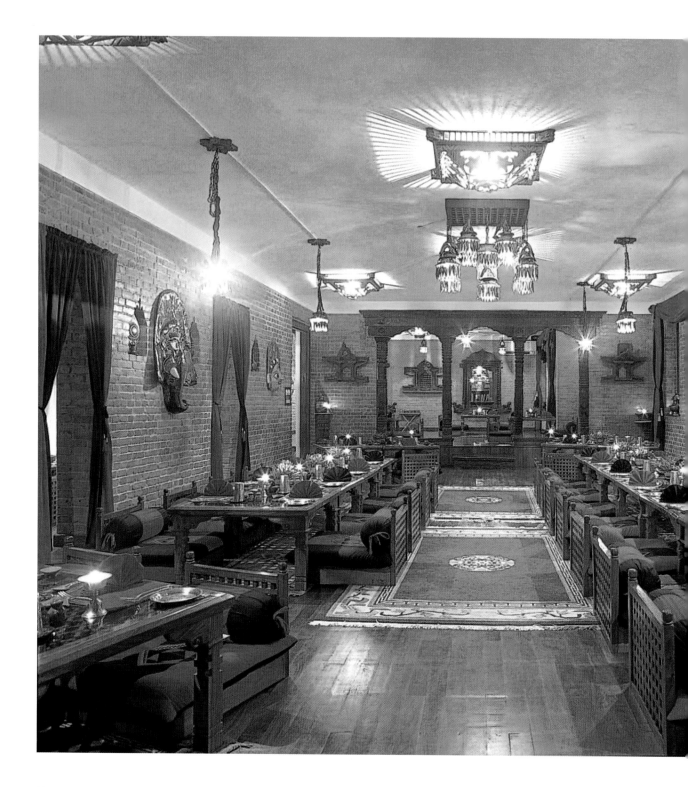

Krishnarpan
restaurant, Nepal

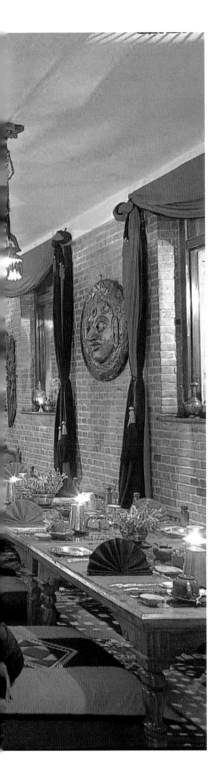

FASHION DESIGNER PRABAL GURUNG ON NEPAL

Nepal sits between two powerful nations—India and Japan—and it embodies and embraces both cultures, but maintains its own strong identity. The landscape of mountains, hills, and plains is stunning and inspiring. It's truly remarkable to have such diversity in a country of its size, between the religions practiced and the languages spoken. My favorite cultural touchstone is the Patan Museum, which is actually an old royal palace with a fantastic Asian art collection. I also love the Garden of Dreams—a magnificent neoclassical garden with pavilions, pergolas, and fountains—because it has such a rich history and is breathtakingly beautiful.

Dining is intimate. There is a strong culture of either going to friends' and families' homes or hosting a dinner and cooking a large meal. I go home for my mother's cooking, so I rarely go to the restaurants. However, Tukuche is great for traditional Nepalese fare and the dishes at Krishnarpan are absolutely exquisite.

For shopping, Thamel Street—also known as "Freak Street"—is where you can buy clothes, crafts, food, and even music. The hippie movement moved through India to Nepal and left such a mark on this street. What to bring home? Pashmina shawls originated in Nepal, so you can never go wrong with one! Also look for a thangka painting, which depicts a Buddhist deity on silk. ∎

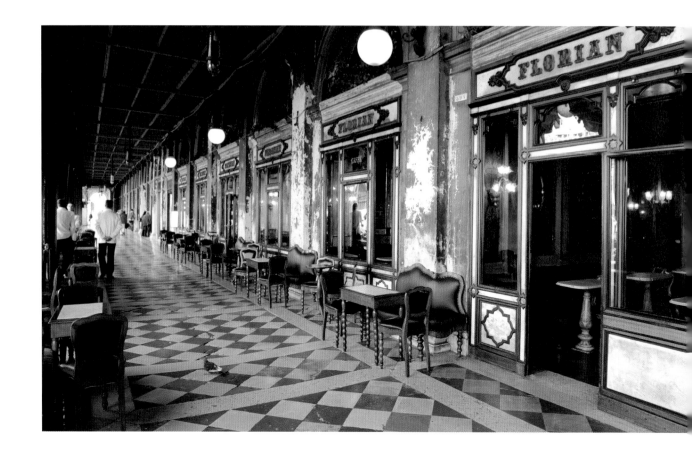

Above: Caffè Florian, Venice.
Opposite: Hotel Danieli, Venice.

PUCCI DESIGNER PETER DUNDAS ON VENICE

As a Norwegian, I love places on the water and Venice is one of my favorite cities. It has to be one of the most romantic places on the planet. A weekend there is an almost guaranteed successful getaway. I usually like to stay at the Hotel Danieli, which is right on the main canal—the sunrises and sunsets are unparalleled. It's nice to sit and have a coffee at Caffè Florian in Piazza San Marco, which opened in 1720. The café sells some of the best home fragrances; Sala Orientale is one of my favorites and it is a staple at my Florence offices.

When it comes to culture, the Fortuny Museum is a well-hidden treasure. It has a great collection of pleated Fortuny delft dresses, a rare editions bookshop, and small exhibitions like one on Roberta di Camerino. Before I leave the city, I make sure to stock up on gold and silver crucifixes from the San Marco Cathedral. I wear them in my ear and seem to lose them in various beds all over the world! It's also one of the best places to buy Murano glass, which is multicolored and reminds me a bit of Pucci patterns. You can find it throughout the city. ■

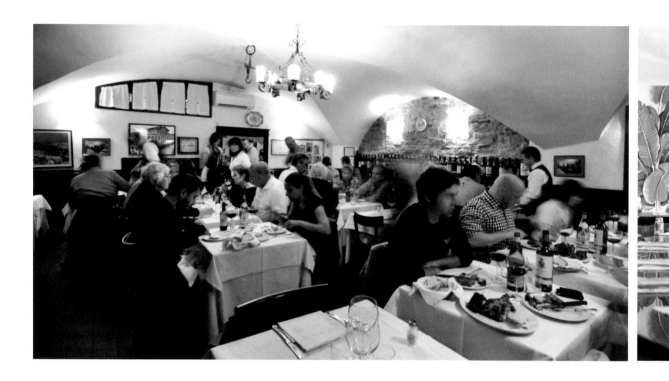

Left: Buca Mario
restaurant, Florence.
Right: Beverly Hills Hotel.

RODARTE DESIGNERS KATE AND LAURA MULLEAVY ON FLORENCE

Florence is one of the most beautiful cities in the world because of its art and architecture. If we have a free morning or afternoon, we always visit the Galleria dell'Accademia di Firenze, which holds Michelangelo's *David* and the unfinished *Prisoners*. Our favorite museum is San Marco, where you can see the Fra Angelico frescoes. We always pick up Botticelli T-shirts as souvenirs!

We love dining at Buca Mario, which opened in 1886 and has an amazing cellar space. For bellinis, we go to Harry's Bar, which overlooks the Arno. They use the most aromatic peaches from northern Italy, and the last time we were there, we received never-ending bowls of the ripest cherries. ∎

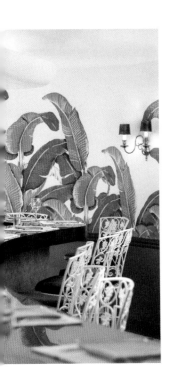

JUICY COUTURE COFOUNDERS PAM SKAIST-LEVY AND GELA NASH TAYLOR ON LOS ANGELES

There is an incredible light that only a sunny day in Los Angeles can bring. It makes you feel like anything is possible and happiness is abounding. Where else can you jump in your car and drive to the sunny shores of Malibu or check out the desert in Two Bunch Palms—just two hours outside the city? There are dozens of great places to stay in the city, but we love the Beverly Hills Hotel. It feels like home because we have been going there our whole lives. When you walk through those doors, you feel like Eloise. Be sure to check out the coffee shop downstairs—it is truly an institution.

For a shot of culture, we are huge fans of the Museum of Contemporary Art (MOCA), which is downtown. It doesn't feel like a corporate museum and never disappoints. We also love its bookstore and gift shop for artsy finds. The funky neighborhood of Echo Park is where you find the most killer vintage shops that have great prices and are well curated. But if you're looking for an authentic souvenir, pick up anything from Olvera Street, which is a historical Mexican marketplace downtown. ■

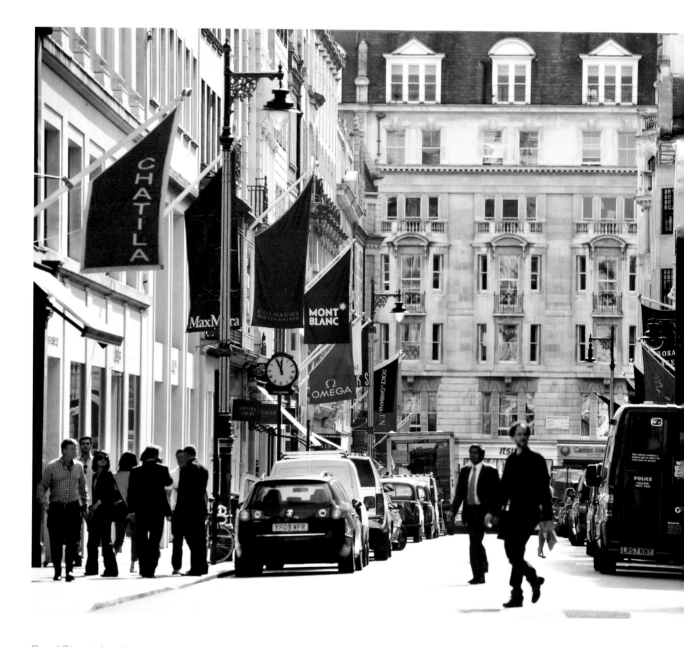

Bond Street, London

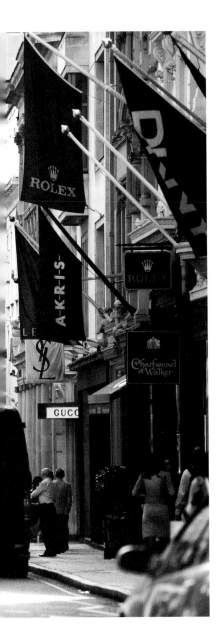

BURBERRY CHIEF CREATIVE OFFICER CHRISTOPHER BAILEY ON LONDON

I am constantly inspired by London on so many levels and I particularly love its people, its architecture, and the wonderful parks and gardens that add green to our city. There's a beautiful hidden English garden in the middle of Battersea Park that is a real gem and gives a moment of calm in the city. You have the well-known, elegant, and bustling shopping areas such as Bond Street, Knightsbridge, and Regent Street—but don't forget to explore the wonderful little streets off the beaten track, too.

When I'm craving culture, I absolutely love the National Portrait Gallery. The portraits take your breath away as they transport you through different periods of time, culture, and politics. Step outside again and you'll find yourself in one of the most bustling, vibrant, and dramatic parts of London: Trafalgar Square. The energy in the air in this part of town simply buzzes.

London is home to some of the best antique bookstores in the world and I like whiling away the hours looking for something special. Try Pottertons in Chelsea for art and design, Peter Harrington on Fulham Road for exquisite and rare first editions, or simply wander along Charing Cross Road and dip into the many bookshops there to bring home a unique reminder of your stay. ■

DESTINATION LUGGAGE

Now that I know about all the hidden gems in these fantastic places, what to bring? Obviously, a week in a cosmopolitan city calls for completely different packing than a jaunt to the slopes. I categorize my trips according to weather, landscape, street style, and activities.

URBAN ESCAPE. City vacations or business trips call for the most versatile clothes and accessories. If you're out all day, you might not want to run back to your hotel to change for dinner. Instead, you can amp up your look with bold jewelry, red lipstick, and heels. For jewelry, think big—or, at least, as big as you can pack. Oversized cuffs can inject texture, color, or a flash of metal to a little black dress or jeans and a tee. I love to top off my metropolitan look with a felt fedora.

When I travel to New York or London, I always bring along a structured bag with a cross-body strap that looks polished but gives me easy, on-the-go access. Cities mean a lot of walking, so cool motorcycle boots or classic riding boots—flat or with a modest wedge or chunky heel—are perfect. Wayfarer sunglasses always feel spot on in the city because they're sleek and architectural.

Denim, skinny or wide in a dark wash, can transition easily from day to night with a pair of platform pumps. A silk button-up blouse also works around the clock—just undo another button and add a statement necklace for an evening out. I like to bring along at least one tuxedo-inspired dress, because it looks androgynously chic in a cosmopolitan setting and also exudes a little rock-and-roll vibe. On windy days or chilly nights, a leather peacoat or bomber jacket is perfect.

BEACH GETAWAY. What I love most about our annual Saint Bart's trip is that I can pack light. If you're heading to a tropical setting or a beach destination, it's all about easy, ethereal pieces like caftans and maxi dresses that mirror the casual vibe. An eyelet sundress that you can wear with gladiator flats during the day or metallic espadrilles at night is key. An oversized raffia tote that can hold my swimsuit, sunscreen, and other beach necessities is my go-to. I like to wear cat-eye sunglasses on the beach, because they make me feel especially glamourous.

Silk harem pants are comfortable and they ripple in a sexy way with a gentle island breeze. Similarly, a printed peasant blouse feels right in line with the atmosphere and pairs well with a lightweight linen blazer. And always be sure to pack a classic black bikini. Jewelry with turquoise, coral, or tiger-eye pops with sun-kissed skin and a bright headscarf or headband is essential for taming an ocean-tousled mane.

WINTER WEEKEND. Cold-weather locales can pose a few packing dilemmas. It's easy to get stuck on shoes when you want to look stylish, but also might encounter ice or snow. My solution is faux fur–lined wedge boots with rubber soles that are both fashionable and functional. They look cute with thick black knit leggings or a cable-knit cashmere sweater dress with a cozy cowl neck.

I opt for a well-worn leather tote or knapsack that can stow a knit beanie and a pair of mirrored aviator sunglasses. You won't have to sacrifice your silhouette, either, in a belted puffer jacket that will keep you warm. Underneath, go with a warm, fitted cashmere sweater and accessorize with an oversized men's watch and quilted leather gloves.

CARRY-ON CHIC

What you bring on a flight in your carry-on bag can make or break the first and last leg of your journey. Over the years, I have learned to pack all my beauty products—from skincare to cosmetics to hair needs—in separate zip pouches so I can stay moisturized in the air and do a quick touch-up before the plane lands. (I transfer certain lotions to three-ounce containers to comply with TSA rules.) I also stash a set in my tote that includes slippers, an eye mask, a small throw, and a miniature pillow. A lot of airlines don't stock enough blankets and pillows for every passenger. You're better off being prepared!

Since checked luggage can often be delayed, I also fold a pair of leggings and a sweater into a pouch so that I have an outfit in a pinch. If I'm heading to the beach, I also include a bathing suit for the same reason. All of my jewelry comes with me in a separate holder, too. Never check valuables, and protect them from scratches by packing each piece in its own velvet pouch. Storing necessary credit cards, airline paperwork, and my passport and license in an accessible zip pocket in my tote makes the process of boarding that much simpler, too. Chargers for tech accessories and sanitizer get pockets as well. Finally, I always pack enough fashion magazines to keep me busy through the entire flight.

AU REVOIR

Well, that was fun! By now, I hope you feel inspired to begin or end your day with more confidence in who you are — or who you want to be. Perhaps you'll spend an extra minute or two in the morning applying a new bold red lipstick or set aside an evening to throw a chic dinner party and tackle a new recipe. Writing this book certainly has reminded me that even a little effort goes a long way.

What I have laid out for you is merely a blueprint. Now, it's your turn to experiment and rewrite the pages. There truly are no rules when it comes to defining your signature style. Be fearless. Trust your creative instincts. Take fashion risks! You only live once — so make every day glamourous.

RACHEL ZOE

Thank you for your tremendous support throughout my career. I hope you enjoyed reading this book as much as I relished working on it. Here's to life, love & endless glamour!

XoRachel Zoe

ACKNOWLEDGMENTS

TEAM ZOE

Monica Corcoran Harel—You are incredibly talented and such a dream to work with! Your enthusiasm and dedication to this book have meant everything to me.

Mandana Dayani—There are not enough words to describe my love and gratitude for who you are and what you mean to me. My friend and my sister, I love you.

Marisa Runyon—It's been a very long road together and I can't thank you enough for always staying by my side and being my champion and my family.

Kelsey Berlacher—You are a star that keeps shining brighter every day. I am eternally grateful to you, my Kels Kels.

Kendall Cohan, Shannon Nash, Jessica Amento, and Mel Chalian—To the greatest team on earth: Thanks for always being my cheerleaders and for making me smile when I didn't think I could. I am forever grateful for your dedication to this project.

Justin Coit—Thank you doesn't say enough for your immeasurable patience and kindness. You always capture the best of me. You are a true friend and my family. You will go so far!

Byron Williams—You are my brother and a genius. I am endlessly grateful to you for helping me find myself.

Joey Maalouf—I cannot thank you enough for always making me feel beautiful and being the most extraordinary uncle to my son. My love for you is immeasurable.

Amanda Englander—Your patience and attention to every page, photo, and very last comma helped shape this book immensely. Thank you!

Andy McNicol—Many thanks for envisioning a follow-up book and convincing me that I had so much more to say.

CONTRIBUTORS

I am so lucky to have such witty, thoughtful, talented, and well-traveled friends who shared their collective brilliance with my readers. Thank you so much for your time and input. You are the everyday inspirations in my life.

Adir Abergel

Brian Atwood

Christopher Bailey

Rodger Berman

Martyn Lawrence Bullard

Francisco Costa

Peter Dundas

Nacho Figueras

Prabal Gurung

Joey Maalouf

Kate Mulleavy

Laura Mulleavy

Leslie Rosenzweig

Ron Rosenzweig

Pam Skaist-Levy

Gela Nash Taylor

Diane von Furstenberg

Matthew Williamson

Beautiful images helped bring this book to life. Thanks to everyone who generously provided art.

Bowery Hotel

Buca Mario

Chanel

Claridge's Hotel

The Cotton House

Didier Ludot

Dorchester Hotel Collection

Dwarika's Hotel

Eric Buterbaugh

Foundation Pierre Berge—Yves Saint Laurent

Four Seasons Hotel George V

Hachette Filipacchi Photos

Hôtel Costes

Hotel Danieli

Hotel Du Cap

La Duree

Le Meurice and Le Dalí

Margherita Missoni and Missoni

Morgans Hotel Group

Nammos

ShoeDazzle

Tiffany & Co.

Tom Ford

Van Cleef & Arpels

RACHEL ZOE

An unparalleled fixture in the fashion world, Rachel Zoe is a distinguished designer, stylist, and editor, renowned for her effortless take on glamour. Having immersed herself in fashion and design for two decades, Rachel has been heralded as one of the most influential forces working in fashion today.

Rachel's first book, *Style A to Zoe*, was published in 2007 and was a *New York Times* bestseller. Very shortly after the success of her book, Rachel debuted *The Rachel Zoe Project* on Bravo in 2008. The show catapulted her from behind-the-scenes stylist to a household name and ran internationally for five successful seasons.

In an effort to further expand her direct relationship with her audience and share her knowledge and expertise, in 2009 Rachel launched *The Zoe Report*, a free daily newsletter featuring her latest obsessions in the ever-evolving worlds of fashion, beauty, and lifestyle. In 2011, she debuted two additional daily newsletters, *Zoe Beautiful* and *AccesZOEries*, focusing on beauty and accessories.

Rachel launched her eponymous contemporary collection in 2011. Drawing on vintage-inspired fabrics, patterns, and the spirit of her style icons from the sixties and seventies, her line introduced separates, footwear, handbags, and jewelry evocative of her modern take on timeless glamour.

Most recently, Rachel co-founded the newly opened chain of blowout salons, DreamDry, launched a television production company, Rachel Zoe Productions, and has aligned with several brands to lend her face, name, and expertise to their initiatives.

She has been the recipient of numerous prestigious industry awards, including The Fashion Group International's Fashion Oracle Award, the Accessories Council Fashion Influencer Ace Award, *Hollywood Life Magazine*'s Star Stylist Award and *Hollywood Reporter*'s Most Influential Stylist. And perhaps most notably, Rachel was the recipient of 2011's Launch of the Year Award from the Footwear News Association and in 2012 was inducted into the Council of Fashion Designers of America (CFDA). She was named Stylist of the Year at the 10th Annual Style Awards at Mercedes-Benz Fashion Week in 2013.

Rachel Zoe currently resides in Los Angeles with her husband and business partner, Rodger Berman, and their sons, Skyler and Kaius.

MONICA CORCORAN HAREL

Monica Corcoran Harel is a writer and consultant who covers fashion, design, and culture. She contributes to the *New York Times*, *ELLE*, *Marie Claire*, *Deadline Hollywood*, and *InStyle*. Her reported essay on cosmetic treatments was part of a 2013 National Magazine Award–winning package for *Los Angeles Magazine*. She has advised on *Project Runway* and co-authored the style book *The Fashion File* with *Mad Men* costume designer Janie Bryant. Corcoran Harel lives in Los Angeles with her husband, Gadi, and their daughter, Tess.

PHOTO CREDITS